Corneal Physiology and
Disposable Contact Lenses

This Book is Presented
in Proud Support

of

WORLDWIDE
CONTACT LENS EDUCATION

Compliments of

VISTAKON™
Division of Johnson & Johnson
Vision Products, Inc.

and its

Johnson & Johnson Affiliates
Worldwide

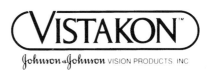

Corneal Physiology and Disposable Contact Lenses

Edited by

Hikaru Hamano, M.D.

Assistant Professor of Ophthalmology, Osaka University Medical School, Suita, Japan; Clinical Professor of Ophthalmology, LSU Eye Center, Louisiana State University Medical Center School of Medicine, New Orleans

Herbert E. Kaufman, M.D.

Boyd Professor of Ophthalmology and Pharmacology and Experimental Therapeutics; Head, Department of Ophthalmology; Director, LSU Eye Center, Louisiana State University Medical Center School of Medicine, New Orleans

Butterworth–Heinemann

Boston   Oxford   Johannesburg   Melbourne   New Delhi   Singapore

Every effort has been made to ensure that the drug dosage schedules within this text are accurate and conform to standards accepted at time of publication. However, as treatment recommendations vary in the light of continuing research and clinical experience, the reader is advised to verify drug dosage schedules herein with information found on product information sheets. This is especially true in cases of new or infrequently used drugs.

Recognizing the importance of preserving what has been written, Butterworth–Heinemann prints its books on acid-free paper whenever possible.

 Butterworth–Heinemann supports the efforts of American Forests and the Global ReLeaf program in its campaign for the betterment of trees, forests, and our environment.

Library of Congress Cataloging-in-Publication Data

Corneal physiology and disposable contact lenses / edited by Hikaru
  Hamano, Herbert E. Kaufman.
        p.   cm.
    Includes bibliographical references and index.
    ISBN 0-7506-9927-2 (alk. paper)
    1. Disposable contact lenses. 2. Cornea--Physiology. I. Hamano,
  Hikaru. II. Kaufman, Herbert E. (Herbert Edward), 1931– .
    [DNLM: 1. Contact Lenses. 2. Cornea--physiology. 3. Disposable
  Equipment.   WW 355 C813 1997]
  RE977.C6C67   1997
  617.7'523--dc21
  DNLM/DLC
  for Library of Congress   97-4330
                                                                        CIP

British Library Cataloguing-in-Publication Data
A catalogue record for this book is available from the British Library.

The publisher offers special discounts on bulk orders of this book.
For information, please contact:

Manager of Special Sales
Butterworth–Heinemann
313 Washington Street
Newton, MA 02158-1626
Tel: 617-928-2500
Fax: 617-928-2620

For information on all B-H medical publications available, contact our World Wide Web home page at: http://www.bh.com/med

10 9 8 7 6 5 4 3 2 1

Printed in the United States of America

To our wives, Ayako Hamano and Maija Kaufman

Contents

Contributing Authors

Roger W. Beuerman, Ph.D.
Professor of Ophthalmology, Anatomy, and Clinical Psychiatry, LSU Eye Center, Louisiana State University Medical Center School of Medicine, New Orleans

Bryan M. Gebhardt, Ph.D.
Professor of Ophthalmology and Microbiology, Parasitology, and Immunology, LSU Eye Center, Louisiana State University Medical Center School of Medicine, New Orleans

Hikaru Hamano, M.D.
Assistant Professor of Ophthalmology, Osaka University Medical School, Suita, Japan; Clinical Professor of Ophthalmology, LSU Eye Center, Louisiana State University Medical Center School of Medicine, New Orleans

Takashi Hamano, M.D.
Assistant Professor of Ophthalmology, Osaka University Medical School, Suita, Japan; Director of Dry Eye Center, Osaka Seamens' Insurance Hospital

Brien A. Holden, Ph.D., D.Sc.
Director, Cornea and Contact Lens Research Unit and The Cooperative Research Centre for Eye Research and Technology, The University of New South Wales, School of Optometry, Sydney, Australia

Herbert E. Kaufman, M.D.
Boyd Professor of Ophthalmology and Pharmacology and Experimental Therapeutics; Head, Department of Ophthalmology; Director, LSU Eye Center, Louisiana State University Medical Center School of Medicine, New Orleans

Stephen D. Klyce, Ph.D.
Professor of Ophthalmology and Anatomy, LSU Eye Center, Louisiana State University Medical Center School of Medicine, New Orleans; Adjunct Professor of Biomedical Engineering, Tulane University, New Orleans

Naoyuki Maeda, M.D.
Assistant Professor of Ophthalmology, Osaka University Medical School, Suita, Japan

George W. Mertz, O.D., F.A.A.O.
Director, Academic Affairs, Vistakon, Division of Johnson & Johnson Vision Products, Inc., Jacksonville, Florida

Claire M. Vajdic, B.Optom.
Manager of Clinical Research, Cornea and Contact Lens Research Unit and The Cooperative Research Centre for Eye Research and Technology, The University of New South Wales, School of Optometry, Sydney, Australia

Kiyoshi Watanabe, M.D.
Assistant Professor of Ophthalmology, Osaka University Medical School, Suita, Japan

Preface

The safety of contact lenses has been a concern to all of us. Hamano and his work have demonstrated that even with highly oxygen-permeable lenses, closure of the lid results in relative oxygen deprivation. In addition, other factors related to lens care can contribute to the risks of contact lens wear. This book illustrates that the use of daily disposable contact lenses can usher in a new era of safety for contact lens–wearing patients and outlines many of the considerations and factors involved in their use.

We would like to thank the chapter authors who contributed their time and effort, as well as their knowledge, to the assembling of this book.

We also acknowledge the efforts of Paula Gebhardt at the editorial office of LSU Eye Center, whose editing and organizational skills made this project possible, and the helpful support of Susan Pioli and Karen Oberheim at Butterworth–Heinemann. Finally, Dr. Hamano thanks Professor Yasuo Tano of Osaka University Medical School and Professor Emeritus Saiichi Mishima of Tokyo University for their continued guidance and encouragement throughout the years.

Hikaru Hamano, M.D.
Herbert E. Kaufman, M.D.

Corneal Physiology and
Disposable Contact Lenses

I

Fundamentals of Corneal Anatomy and Physiology

1

Functional Anatomy of the Cornea*

Roger W. Beuerman, Stephen D. Klyce, and
Herbert E. Kaufman

The cornea is a transparent tissue consisting of three layers, two membranes, and
three major types of cells (Figure 1.1). The cornea protects the inner ocular structures and contributes approximately 70% of the refractive power of the eye.

On the anterior, outermost surface of the cornea is the epithelium, comprising
five to seven layers of cells (Teng 1961; Hogan et al. 1971; Kuwabara 1978;
Klyce and Beuerman 1988). The basal layer of epithelial cells is attached to the
basement membrane, and the basement membrane is apposed directly to Bowman's layer, which forms the anterior margin of the stroma. The stroma makes
up the bulk of the corneal tissue; most of the stroma is extracellular matrix, with
only a few cells—the keratocytes—interspersed among the collagen fibrils. The
posterior surface of the stroma is limited by Descemet's membrane, a basement
membrane secreted by the endothelial cells. A single layer of endothelial cells
lines the posterior surface, forming a barrier between the cornea and the fluid-
filled anterior chamber.

The cornea is slightly oval; as a rule, in approximately 90% of eyes, the vertical
dimension is the short axis (with-the-rule), and the longer axis is the horizontal dimension (against-the-rule). Normal corneal thickness is approximately 0.50–0.57
mm in the central optical zone and 0.85–0.90 mm in the periphery. The radius of
curvature of the normal cornea averages 7.8 mm. Free nerve endings are located
between the corneal epithelial cells, where they sense virtually all stimuli as pain.
The cornea is an avascular tissue; the appearance of blood vessels in the cornea
generally indicates some abnormal irritation or disease process.

THE EPITHELIUM AND THE BASEMENT MEMBRANE

The corneal epithelium is a self-renewing, protective layer of cells that provides
the interface between the cornea and the environment (Segawa 1964; Klyce and

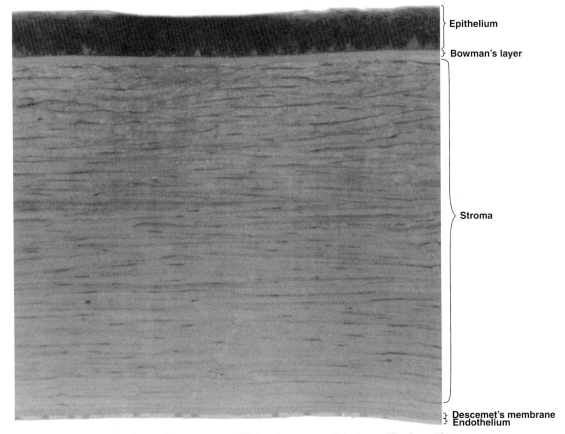

Epithelium

Bowman's layer

Stroma

Descemet's membrane
Endothelium

Figure 1.1 Cross-section of normal human cornea. (Light microscope; original magnification ×46.)

Beuerman 1988). Most of the refraction of the eye occurs at the air–cornea interface,* and the regularity of this interface is primarily responsible for the clarity of
the focused image on the retina. Any distortion, no matter how slight, can degrade
the retinal image greatly, and irregular astigmatism frequently is underestimated as
a primary cause of poor vision.

The surface of the outermost epithelial cells is not keratinized but is covered with
a network of microscopic ridges called *microvilli* (Hoffman 1972; Pfister 1973) (Figure 1.2). These irregularities are thought to increase the surface area and to provide
a roughened surface that aids in the adherence of the tear film and prevents drying
(Pfister and Renner 1977; Nichols et al. 1983).

The outermost layer is made up of flattened, overlapping cells; the layers beneath
become progressively more columnar in shape (Figures 1.3 and 1.4). The internal
borders of the epithelial cells have projections and infoldings, and the cells are "spot-

---

*Actually, most of the refraction occurs at the air–tear interface, but for the purposes of this text, we will
consider them synonymous.

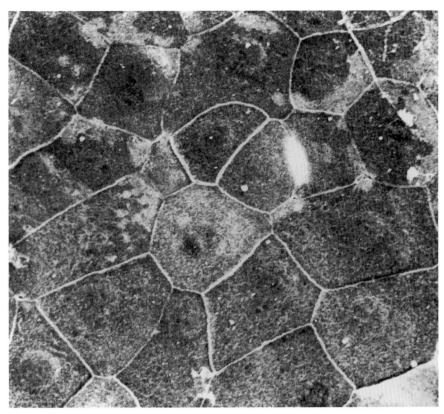

Figure 1.2 Scanning electron micrograph of human corneal epithelium. (Original magnification ×1,000.)

welded" together at intervals along these interdigitations by desmosomes (maculae adherens) (Klyce and Beuerman 1988) (Figure 1.5).

The tight junctions of the surface or squamous cells prevent the entry of noxious materials from the tears and prevent overhydration of the cornea by fluid from the tears. If these tight junctions are damaged, the stroma can imbibe fluid focally, leading to edema (Kikkawa 1972). The layers beneath—the wing and basal cells— are less tightly joined, permitting the movement of fluid from the stroma into the epithelium. The tight junctions prevent bulk flow of fluid from the endothelial surface through the cornea and into the tear film, however, so that when excess fluid enters the cornea—by the force of high intraocular pressure as in acute glaucoma or by normal pressure in the eye in the face of a defective endothelial barrier—it accumulates under the seal and results in epithelial edema (Hedbys et al. 1963; Klyce et al. 1971).

The basal layer of epithelial cells is a single layer of columnar cells that makes up slightly less than half the thickness of the epithelium. The mitotic activity that replaces the epithelial cell population takes place in these cells; as new cells are produced, the older cells migrate toward the surface, lose their columnar shape, and eventually are sloughed as debris in the tears. It has become clear that the basal epithelium is not uniform in its mitotic potential. The limbal epithelium seems to have much greater capacity for mitosis and healing and is considered by some to be a

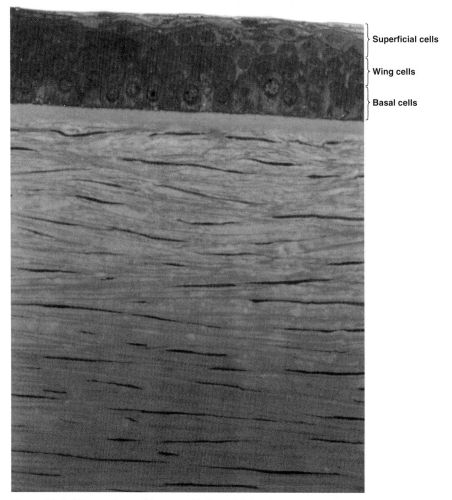

Superficial cells

Wing cells

Basal cells

Figure 1.3 Cell layers of normal human epithelium. (Light microscope; original magnification ×63.)

"stem cell" area. If the epithelium is removed or damaged, the resurfacing of the cornea is improved dramatically if limbal epithelial cells are retained. Because of the multilayer structure of the corneal epithelium, however, it is possible to heal epithelial defects several millimeters in diameter by sliding of the cells so that mitotic function takes place in the area around the defect (Thompson et al. 1991).

The contents of the epithelial cells include tonofilaments in the columnar cells, as well as glycogen granules, rough endoplasmic reticulum, ribosomes, and a few small mitochondria (Hogan et al. 1971; Kuwabara 1978; Klyce and Beuerman 1988). Under anaerobic conditions, such as the hypoxia present with some kinds of contact lenses, excess lactic acid may be produced (Klyce 1981; Hamano et al. 1983). The presence of the lactic acid causes an inflow of water, resulting in epithelial and stromal edema, and may be responsible for the presence of blebs in the endothelium, which are seen acutely when oxygen-impermeable contact lenses are placed on the surface of the cornea (Bonanno and Polse 1987).

The posterior surface of the basal epithelial cells is flattened and is attached to the basement membrane beneath by hemidesmosomes which, as the name implies,

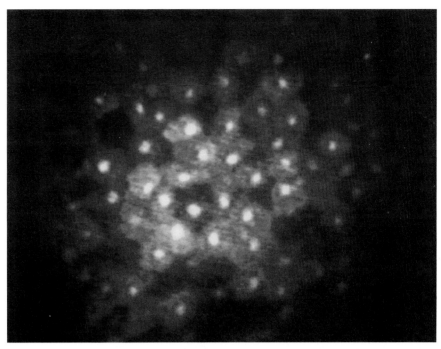

Figure 1.4 Real-time confocal micrograph of the outermost cell layer of the living human corneal epithelium in vivo, showing the layer of contiguous cells with prominent nuclei. (Original magnification ×230.)

look like one-half of a desmosome (Tisdale et al. 1988). The basement membrane, which is approximately 65 nm thick, is secreted by the basal epithelial cells and is directly adjacent to Bowman's layer, the anterior surface of the corneal stroma. Overproduction of basement membrane can result in map-dot-fingerprint dystrophies and recurrent erosions because the epithelium tends to attach poorly to this abnormal basement membrane (Azar et al. 1992). Removal of the basement membrane, either mechanically or with an excimer laser, often can restore normal epithelial adhesion. Similarly, alkali and other chemical injuries also may denature the basement membrane and interfere with epithelial hemidesmosomal attachment.

BOWMAN'S LAYER AND THE STROMA

Bowman's layer is approximately 170 times the thickness of the epithelial basement membrane. By light microscopy, it appears to be a distinct layer in the superficial stroma, but electron microscopy has demonstrated that Bowman's layer actually is part of the stroma, with only slight structural modifications (Klyce and Beuerman 1988). There are no cells in Bowman's layer. The fibrils are aggregated into short fibers that are not ordered, as they are in the deeper stroma.

The origin of Bowman's layer is unknown; it is found only in primates and in certain fowl, reptiles, and elasmobranchs (Hay 1980). The characteristic structure does not regenerate if it is disorganized or destroyed by pathologic processes or surgical intervention. Natural disruption of the integrity of Bowman's layer is rare, but

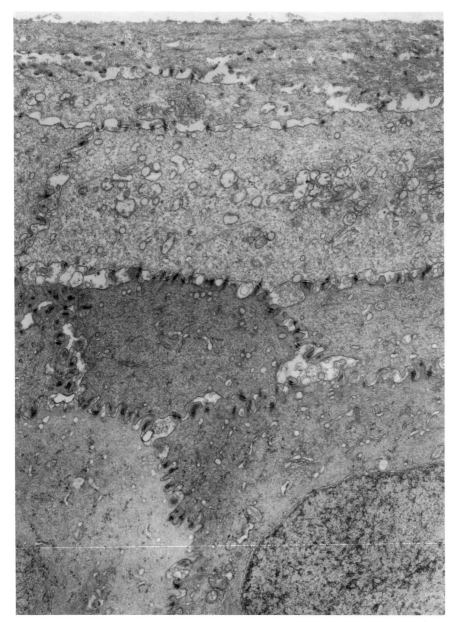

Figure 1.5 Transmission electron micrograph of the upper layers of human corneal epithelium. The flattening of the cells as they move from the wing cell level toward the surface is particularly obvious. Numerous desmosomal contacts are visible as small, dense bands extending across the membranes of adjacent cells. (Original magnification ×11,000.)

when it occurs in the optical zone, as in trauma or keratoconus, the resulting irregularity degrades vision in proportion to the amount of irregular astigmatism induced. Surprisingly, when Bowman's layer is removed by means of excimer laser ablation, healing can occur without such irregularities. Because most laboratory animals lack Bowman's layer, experimental studies of corneal warpage and changes in corneal shape with refractive surgery usually are not applicable to humans.

In the stroma, the diameter of the collagen fibrils is approximately 340–400 Å. The fibrils are arranged in orderly layers attached at both ends at the limbus (Maurice 1984). All the layers are oriented parallel to the corneal surface, but they course in different directions such that a cross-section shows some layers of fibrils perpendicular to the long axis of the cornea, other layers parallel to the long axis, and still others at various angles in between. With this arrangement of regularly spaced, crisscrossing fibrils, the cornea can be both strong and transparent, to serve both protective and optical functions. This arrangement of the fibrils also makes possible the lamellar splitting of the cornea, as it divides the stroma into loosely connected, relatively distinct planes that can be separated without difficulty by blunt dissection.

The stroma is made up largely of extracellular matrix, including the collagen fibrils, other proteins, and glycosaminoglycans (mucopolysaccharides), and it is approximately 78% water (Cintron et al. 1973; Yue et al. 1978; Maurice 1984). Keratan sulfate, chondroitin, and chondroitin sulfate are the large molecules that play an essential role in corneal hydration in terms of their interactions with electrolytes and water. The only cell type indigenous to the stroma is the keratocyte. These connective tissue cells are large and flat and are scattered sparsely between the collagen lamellae, with contiguous and interdigitated projections. Other freely moving cells seen in the stroma include histiocytes, lymphocytes, and occasional polymorphonuclear leukocytes. These cells generally are present in response to some abnormal condition, and there is some disagreement as to whether they can be seen as normal residents of a healthy cornea.

The clarity of the stroma is critical for good vision. Dense opacities that do not occlude the entrance pupil completely usually cause little degradation of vision, however, and it is easy to overestimate their potential effect on vision. Generally, the primary causes of visual disturbance are irregularities of the anterior or posterior refracting surfaces of the cornea in the absence of total opacification of the visual axis.

DESCEMET'S MEMBRANE AND THE ENDOTHELIUM

Lining the inner curve of the cornea and separating it from the anterior chamber are the corneal endothelium and its basement membrane, called *Descemet's membrane* (Kuwabara 1978; Klyce and Beuerman 1988) (Figure 1.6). Descemet's membrane is approximately 10 μm thick and is secreted by the endothelial cells. The anterior portion of the membrane, which is contiguous to the stroma, is fibrous and banded, whereas the posterior portion adjacent to the endothelial cells is a more homogeneous, nonbanded granular material. Descemet's membrane is elastic and recovers quickly after deformation; however, disease processes can rupture Descemet's membrane. The broken membrane tends to curl inward and is not repaired, but new membranelike material is laid down on the bare stroma by the invading fibroblastic endothelial cells.

Descemet's membrane is elaborated by "activated" endothelial cells. As endothelial cells die with age and others move to take their place, Descemet's membrane is produced. Descemet's membrane therefore increases throughout life (Johnson et al. 1982; Alvarado et al. 1983). Corneal diseases that damage the endothelium, such as deep interstitial keratitis or corneal macular dystrophy, generally result in excessive production of basement membrane or cornea guttata, or both (Burns et al. 1981). In some older people, the thickening of basement membrane may not be uniform, and guttae are seen as a sign of endothelial cell dysfunction.

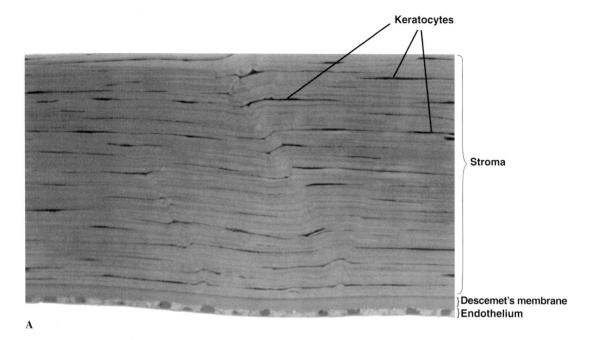

Keratocytes

Stroma

} **Descemet's membrane**
} **Endothelium**

A

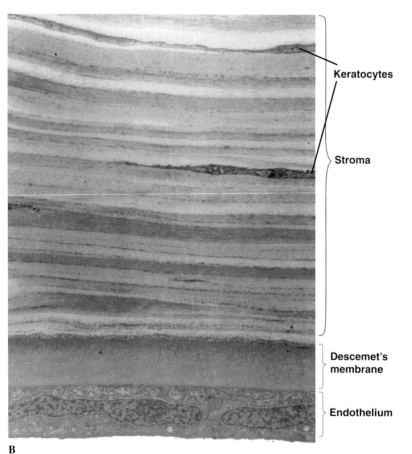

Keratocytes

Stroma

Descemet's membrane

Endothelium

B

Figure 1.6 A. Light micrograph of posterior stroma and endothelial cell layer in the human cornea. (Original magnification ×75.) B. Low-power transmission electron micrograph of the posterior stroma and endothelium. The stroma has its usual banded appearance. In the posterior stroma, the collagen lamellae tend to be somewhat more regular in thickness. Keratocyte processes are seen lying along the interface between adjacent lamellae. Descemet's membrane, the basement membrane of the endothelium, provides a substrate for the endothelium. (Original magnification ×6,000.)

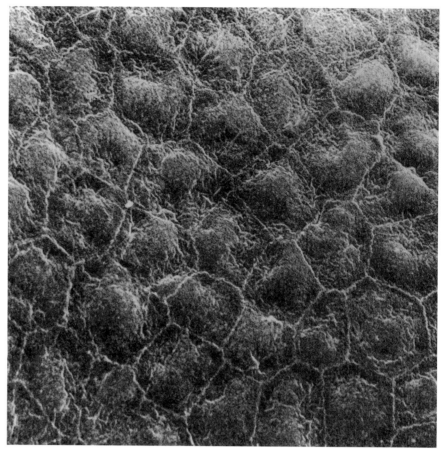

Figure 1.7 Scanning electron micrograph of human corneal endothelium. (Original magnification ×1,300.)

The endothelial cells are flat and hexagonal, and they seem to pave the posterior surface of the cornea with a single layer of cells that are in direct contact with the aqueous humor (Laing et al. 1975; Kreutziger 1976) (Figures 1.7 and 1.8). The endothelial cells have tight junctions between them, but the layer as a whole is characterized as "leaky," allowing water and nutrients to move into the cornea and maintaining stromal hydration by active salt transport. These cells have large numbers of mitochondria, indicating the high energy needed to maintain the endothelial pump that keeps the cornea dehydrated and transparent (Maurice 1968; McCartney et al. 1987). In humans, there is little or no endothelial cell division, and coverage of the posterior cornea is maintained by the enlarging and spreading of existing cells to fill in where cells have been lost (Figure 1.9). Endothelial cells are lost as a natural consequence of aging and as a result of trauma, damage during surgery, or disease (Bourne and Brubaker 1983). When there are too few endothelial cells to cover Descemet's membrane, the barrier function fails; water enters the stroma from the aqueous humor and is not pumped out again. The resulting stromal edema is a major cause of decreased vision and the need for cornea transplantation in older individuals. Because the endothelial cells cannot replace themselves, normal stromal hydration can be re-

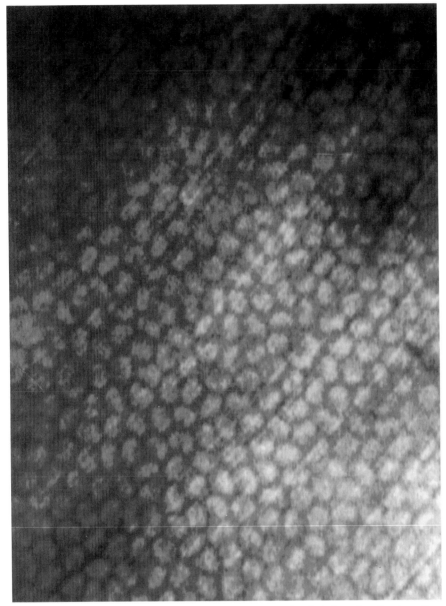

Figure 1.8 Real-time confocal microscopy of the human corneal endothelium showing the cellular morphology and the single, continuous layer of cells. (Original magnification ×230.)

stored only when the defective tissue is replaced by a donor cornea that has adequate endothelial coverage.

INNERVATION OF THE CORNEA

Corneal sensitivity is mediated by free nerve endings situated among the cells of the epithelial layer (Figure 1.10). The axons from these sensory elements form the long

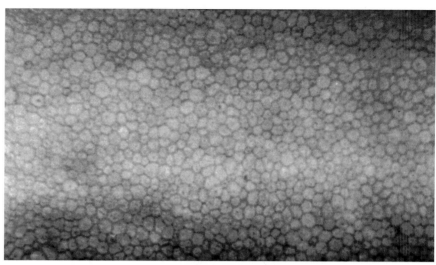

Figure 1.9 Specular micrograph of normal endothelium of human cornea. (Reprinted with permission from H Hamano, HE Kaufman. The Physiology of the Cornea and Contact Lens Applications. New York: Churchill Livingstone, 1987;8.)

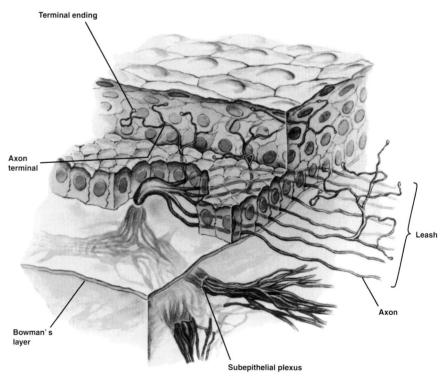

Figure 1.10 Graphic illustration of corneal nerves. (Adapted and redrawn from AJ Rózsa, RW Beuerman. Density and organization of free nerve endings in the corneal epithelium of the rabbit. Pain 1982;14:105.)

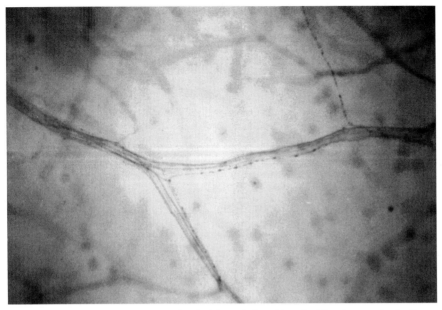

Figure 1.11 A large stromal nerve stained with methylene blue. In this micrograph, the limbus is just out of the picture on the right side. Individual axons within this large nerve have taken up stain and can be followed past the first branch point (×250). (Courtesy of Dr. Roger W. Beuerman, New Orleans, LA. Reprinted with permission from H Hamano, HE Kaufman. The Physiology of the Cornea and Contact Lens Applications. New York: Churchill Livingstone, 1987;11.)

ciliary nerves and contribute to the short ciliary nerves, whereas their cell bodies lie in the rostral portion of the trigeminal ganglion.

Twelve to 16 large, radially oriented nerve branches enter the cornea at the mid-stromal level at various clock positions around the limbus (Rózsa and Beuerman 1982) (Figure 1.11). As these nerves course toward the center of the cornea, they branch horizontally and vertically, forming the dense subepithelial plexus beneath Bowman's layer. From this plexus, axonal extensions pass through Bowman's layer and into the epithelium by means of openings in the basal lamina. All nerve fibers carry an investment of Schwann cells, although processes from one Schwann cell may envelop several axons. Most axons of the corneal nerves are unmyelinated, even at the limbus, and those that are myelinated lose this covering within 2–3 mm of the limbus. On the other hand, all nerve fibers are protected by Schwann cells up to the point of their interaction with the basal lamina as they enter the epithelium (Matsuda 1967).

Only the intraepithelial nerve terminal (Figure 1.12) has the ability to transmit sensory stimuli. These nerve terminals branch at all levels within the corneal epithelium. Although they are most numerous at the basal wing cell level, some reach within one to two cells of the tear layer. Virtually all sensory stimuli that impinge on the cornea are sensed as irritation or pain by the corneal nerves (Beuerman et al. 1985).

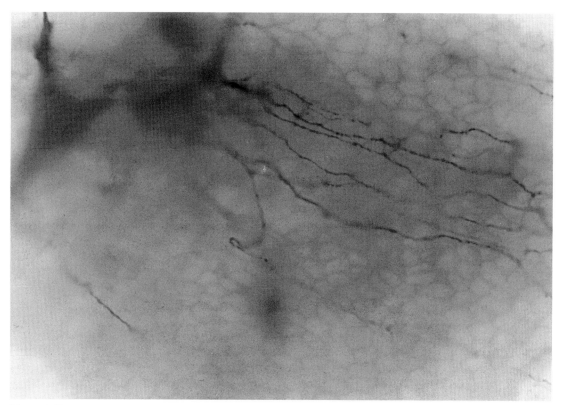

Figure 1.12 Intraepithelial nerve terminals and subepithelial plexus stained by the gold chloride technique. A nerve is seen entering the epithelium and giving rise to several fine terminals. The cornea is mounted flat, and the faint outline of the basal cells can be seen (×400). (Courtesy of Dr. Roger W. Beuerman, New Orleans, LA. Reprinted with permission from H Hamano, HE Kaufman. The Physiology of the Cornea and Contact Lens Applications. New York: Churchill Livingstone, 1987;11.)

REFERENCES

Alvarado J, Murphy C, Juster R. Age-related changes in the basement membrane of the human corneal epithelium. Invest Ophthalmol Vis Sci 1983;24:1015.

Azar DT, Spurr-Michaud SJ, Tisdale AS, Gibson IK. Altered epithelial-basement membrane interactions in diabetic corneas. Arch Ophthalmol 1992;110:537.

Beuerman RW, Rózsa AJ, Tanelian DL. Neurophysiological Correlates of Posttraumatic Acute Pain. In HL Fields, R Dubner, F Cervero (eds), Advances in Pain Research and Therapy, Vol. 9. New York: Raven, 1985;73.

Bonanno JA, Polse KA. Corneal acidosis during contact lens wear: effects of hypoxia and CO_2. Invest Ophthalmol Vis Sci 1987;28:1514.

Bourne WM, Brubaker RF. Decreased endothelial permeability in transplanted corneas. Am J Ophthalmol 1983;96:362.

Burns RR, Bourne WM, Brubaker RF. Endothelial function in patients with cornea guttata. Invest Ophthalmol Vis Sci 1981;20:77.

Cintron C, Schneider H, Kublin C. Corneal scar formation. Exp Eye Res 1973;17:251.

Hamano H, Hori M, Hamano T, et al. Effect of contact lens wear on the mitosis of corneal epithelial cells and the amount of lactate in aqueous humor. Jpn J Ophthalmol 1983;27:451.

Hay ED. Development of the vertebrate cornea. Int Rev Cytol 1980;61:263.

Hedbys BO, Mishima S, Maurice DM. The imbibition pressure of the corneal stroma. Exp Eye Res 1963;2:99.

Hoffman F. The surface of epithelial cells of the cornea under the scanning electron microscope. Ophthalmic Res 1972;3:207.

Hogan MJ, Alvarado JA, Weddell E. Histology of the Human Eye. Philadelphia: Saunders, 1971.

Johnson DH, Bourne WM, Campbell RJ. The ultrastructure of Descemet's membrane: I. Changes with age in normal corneas. Arch Ophthalmol 1982;100:1942.

Kikkawa Y. Normal corneal staining with fluorescein. Exp Eye Res 1972;14:13.

Klyce SD. Stromal lactate accumulation can account for corneal edema osmotically following epithelial hypoxia in the rabbit. J Physiol 1981;321:49.

Klyce SD, Beuerman RW. Structure and Function of the Cornea. In HE Kaufman, BA Barron, MB McDonald, SR Waltman (eds), The Cornea. New York: Churchill Livingstone, 1988;3.

Klyce SD, Dohlman CH, Tolpin DW. In vivo determination of corneal swelling pressure of the corneal stroma. Exp Eye Res 1971;11:220.

Kreutziger GO. Lateral membrane morphology and gap junction structure in rabbit corneal endothelium. Exp Eye Res 1976;23:285.

Kuwabara T. Current concepts in anatomy and histology of the cornea. Contact Intraocul Lens Med J 1978;4:101.

Laing RA, Sandstrom MA, Liebowitz HM. In vivo photomicrography of corneal endothelium. Arch Ophthalmol 1975;93:143.

Matsuda H. Electron microscopic study on the corneal nerve with special reference to its endings. Jpn J Ophthalmol 1967;12:163.

Maurice DM. Cellular membrane activity in the corneal endothelium of the intact eye. Experientia 1968;24:1094.

Maurice DM. The Cornea and Sclera. In H Davson (ed), The Eye, Vol. 1B: Vegetative Physiology and Biochemistry (3rd ed). New York: Academic, 1984;1.

McCartney MD, Robertson DP, Wood TO, McLaughlin BJ. ATPase pump site density in human dysfunctional corneal endothelium. Invest Ophthalmol Vis Sci 1987;28:1955.

Nichols B, Dawson CR, Togni B. Surface features of the conjunctiva and cornea. Invest Ophthalmol Vis Sci 1983;24:570.

Pfister RR. The normal surface of corneal epithelium: a scanning and electron microscopic study. Invest Ophthalmol 1973;12:654.

Pfister R, Renner M. The histopathology of experimental dry spots and dellen in the rabbit cornea: a light microscopy and scanning and transmission electron microscopy study. Invest Ophthalmol Vis Sci 1977;16:1025.

Rózsa AJ, Beuerman RW. Density and organization of free nerve endings in the corneal epithelium of the rabbit. Pain 1982;14:105.

Segawa K. Electron microscopic studies on the human corneal epithelium: dendritic cells. Arch Ophthalmol 1964;72:650.

Teng CC. The fine structure of the corneal epithelium and basement membrane of the rabbit. Am J Ophthalmol 1961;51:278.

Thompson HE, Malter JM, Steinemann TL, Beuerman RW. Flow cytometry measurements of the DNA content of corneal epithelial cells during wound healing. Invest Ophthalmol Vis Sci 1991;32:433.

Tisdale AS, Spurr-Michaud SJ, Rodrigues M, et al. Development of the anchoring structures of the epithelium in rabbit and human fetal corneas. Invest Ophthalmol Vis Sci 1988;29:727.

Yue BYJT, Baum JL, Silbert JE. Synthesis of glycosaminoglycans by cultures of normal human corneal endothelial and stromal cells. Invest Ophthalmol Vis Sci 1978;17:523.

2

Oxygen Permeability of Contact Lenses and Corneal Physiology

Hikaru Hamano

OXYGEN TENSION

When the cornea is covered with a contact lens, one of the first concerns is to maintain an adequate supply of oxygen. Therefore, direct measurement of the oxygen level under the lens (i.e., actual oxygen tension [PO_2] on the cornea) is essential in evaluating the oxygen permeability of contact lenses in vivo.

The oxygen permeability of a contact lens commonly is described in terms of the rate of oxygen flow through a given area of the material. This rate is called the *Dk* and generally is given as a whole number $\times 10^{-11}$ (cm^2/sec) • (ml O_2/ml • mm Hg). A second and similar parameter, oxygen transmissibility, defines both rate of flow and thickness of the material and is given as *Dk/L*, where *L* is the thickness. In this chapter, Dk is used to describe the oxygen permeability of a given contact lens; the higher the Dk, the more permeable the lens is to oxygen.

Hamano et al. (1984, 1986a,b) used a PO_2 monitoring system with a platinum microelectrode to measure oxygen tension in rabbit eyes and in human subjects with and without contact lenses and with open and closed eyelids.

In a preliminary experiment, PO_2 was measured in vivo in the aqueous humor and the conjunctival sac of rabbit eyes without contact lenses. In the aqueous humor, PO_2 ranged from 16 to 45 mm Hg, with an average of 31 mm Hg. In the conjunctival sac, the range was 26–53 mm Hg, and the average was approximately 39 mm Hg. These values are considerably lower than the generally accepted value of 55 mm Hg.

To determine the effect of contact lens wear, PO_2 also was measured simultaneously on the surface of the cornea and in the stroma of enucleated rabbit eyes wearing polymethyl methacrylate (PMMA) hard contact lenses and rigid gas-permeable contact lenses (Figure 2.1). Ten minutes of PMMA lens wear (Dk = 0) reduced the PO_2 to zero, both on the cornea and in the stroma. With a rigid gas-permeable lens having a Dk of 13×10^{-11}, however, the reduction in PO_2 was less steep, and the PO_2 fell to a low of only approximately 20 mm Hg. Rigid gas-permeable lenses with higher Dks (61, 108, and 165×10^{-11}) also produced reductions in PO_2, but the higher the Dk, the smaller the drop in PO_2.

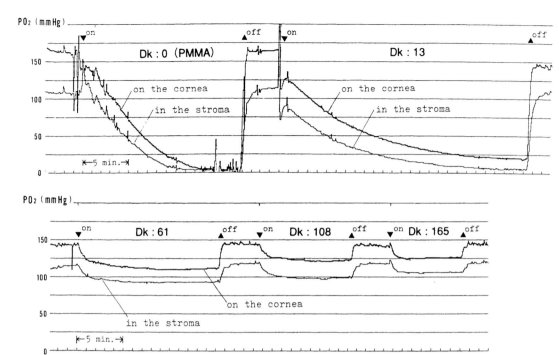

Figure 2.1 Simultaneous measurements of oxygen tension (PO_2) on the cornea and in the stroma of an enucleated rabbit eye wearing a polymethyl methacrylate (PMMA) contact lens or one of four rigid gas-permeable lenses with different oxygen permeabilities (Dk). Lens thickness is 0.13 mm. Dk units are $\times 10^{-11}$ (cm²/sec) • (ml O_2/ml • mm Hg). (Reprinted with permission from H Hamano. Contact lens wear and corneal physiology. J Jpn Contact Lens Soc 1985;27:145.)

In later experiments, PO_2 was measured in vivo on rabbit corneas wearing various kinds of contact lenses, including hard lenses with different oxygen permeabilities (Figure 2.2) and hydrophilic soft lenses with different water contents and thicknesses (Figure 2.3). The greater the oxygen permeability or water content of the lens, the higher the PO_2 under the lens. With soft lenses of the same water content, the thinner the lens, the higher the PO_2 on the cornea. The highest PO_2 (105 mm Hg) was measured under a silicone elastomer lens with a thickness of 0.16 mm (data not shown).

Similar measurements were made with the eyelids closed (see Figures 2.2 and 2.3). Generally, it is accepted that the PO_2 on the cornea with no lens and closed eyelids is 55 mm Hg. With the various lenses in place under closed eyelids, however, PO_2 was reduced markedly, ranging from approximately 5 to 20 mm Hg depending on the type of lens.

Finally, the same technique was applied to human eyes wearing the same kinds of lenses. In these eyes, PO_2 in the conjunctival sac ranged from 23 to 46 mm Hg; the average was approximately 34 mm Hg. The PO_2 under each type of lens was essentially similar to that seen in the rabbit eyes.

Figure 2.2 Oxygen tension (PO_2) on rabbit corneas under hard contact lenses with different oxygen permeabilities (Dk) and eyelids open or closed. The thickness of the rigid gas-permeable lenses was 0.13 mm. Dk units are $\times 10^{-11}$ (cm^2/sec) • (ml O_2/ml • mm Hg). Values plotted are means and standard deviations of six to nine eyes. (PMMA = polymethyl methacrylate; RGP = rigid gas-permeable.)

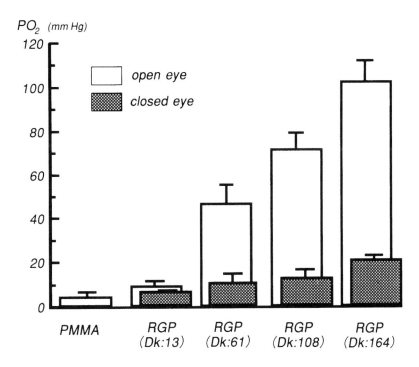

Figure 2.3 Oxygen tension (PO_2) on rabbit corneas under soft contact lenses with different water contents and thicknesses and eyelids open or closed. Values plotted are means and standard deviations of four to seven eyes.

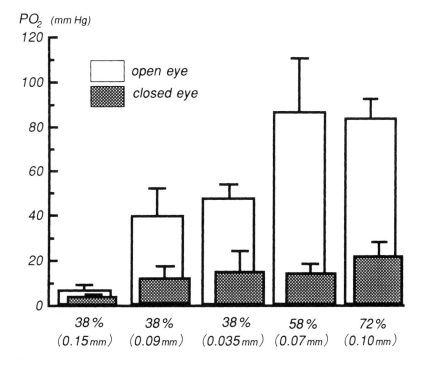

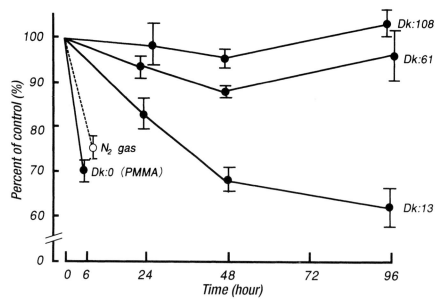

Figure 2.4 Changes in numbers of mitotic figures counted in basal epithelial cell layer during polymethyl methacrylate (PMMA) and rigid gas-permeable lens wear. The thickness of the rigid gas-permeable lenses was 0.13 mm. Value labeled N_2 gas represents eyes with no lenses wearing goggles containing only nitrogen gas. For each time interval, the data from six rabbits were averaged, and the ratios of the number of mitotic figures in the experimental eyes to the number in the controls were computed and expressed as percentage of control (no lens wear). Oxygen permeability (*Dk*) units are $\times 10^{-11}$ (cm²/sec) • (ml O_2/ml • mm Hg). (Reprinted with permission from H Hamano. Contact lens wear and corneal physiology. J Jpn Contact Lens Soc 1985;27:145.)

EPITHELIAL CELL DIVISION

Cell division is characteristic of the normal corneal epithelium, and mitotic configurations are numerous in the basal epithelial cell layer. The rate of mitosis is reduced when there is a deficiency in the amount of available oxygen, however.

Hamano et al. (1983) examined the metabolic effects of oxygen supply through hard contact lenses in terms of the numbers of mitotic figures in the epithelium of rabbit eyes wearing PMMA lenses and three types of rigid gas-permeable lenses. Each type of lens was placed on one eye of a rabbit, with the fellow eye used as the control. To examine the effect of a completely oxygen-free state, goggles with circulating nitrogen gas were used.

Figure 2.4 compares epithelial mitosis under three different conditions: PMMA lens wear, rigid gas-permeable lens wear, and nitrogen gas environment with no contact lens. The effect of a PMMA lens on epithelial mitosis is similar to that of nitrogen gas circulation in the goggles; the number of mitotic figures is reduced sharply under both of these conditions. With rigid gas-permeable lenses, the degree of mitotic suppression is related inversely to the Dk value of the lens. That is, the higher the oxygen permeability (i.e., the higher the PO_2 on the cornea under the lens), the less suppression of cell division is seen. A lens with a Dk value of 108×10^{-11}, which maintained a PO_2 of approximately 70 mm Hg on the cornea (see Figure 2.2), could remain on the cornea for as long as 96 hours with little or no effect on the rate of epithelial mitosis (see Figure 2.4).

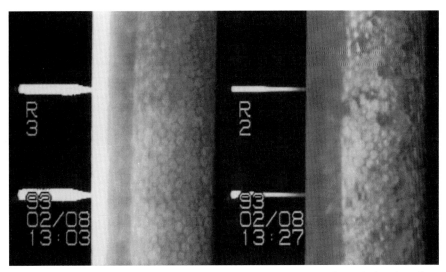

Figure 2.5 Endothelial bleb formation induced by 38%-water-content hydroxyethyl methacrylate lens with thickness of 0.15 mm. Left. Baseline. Right. After 20 minutes of lens wear. The distance between the parallel bars to the left of each image represents 0.2 mm. (Reprinted with permission from H Hamano, K Watanabe, S Mitsunaga. Observation of corneal endothelial response to hydrogel lenses by non-contact specular microscope [TOPCON SP-1000]. J Jpn Contact Lens Soc 1993;35:140.)

ENDOTHELIAL BLEB FORMATION

Zantos and Holden (1977) were the first to describe transient dark areas that developed in the corneal endothelium within minutes after the placement of a soft contact lens in patients who previously had not worn contact lenses. The authors referred to these dark areas, which were as large as a few cells in width, as *endothelial blebs*. Since then, more detailed observations by other researchers (Barr and Schoessler 1980; Schoessler et al. 1982; Efron et al. 1984; Holden et al. 1985; Williams and Holden 1986) have shown that the blebs appear 5–15 minutes after soft lens placement. The number of blebs reaches a maximum at 30 minutes and then gradually decreases. In most cases, the blebs vanish entirely within approximately 90 minutes. Bleb formation commonly is believed to be an acute, transient reaction to corneal hypoxia. The blebs appear to be caused by the development of edema in parts of the endothelial cell mosaic (Vannas et al. 1984; Efron and Holden 1986).

Recently, Hamano et al. (1993) used a noncontact specular microscope with autoshutter function to observe the bleb phenomenon in 22 eyes of 11 patients with no history of contact lens wear. Five kinds of soft contact lenses were used: three types of 38%-water-content hydroxyethyl methacrylate (HEMA) lenses with different thicknesses (0.15, 0.09, and 0.035 mm), a 58%-water-content lens (0.07 mm), and a 72%-water-content lens (0.15 mm). Images were obtained before the insertion of the lens and after 20 minutes of wear. In cases in which the lens alone did not induce bleb formation, the effect of closing the eyelids over the lens for 20 minutes also was examined.

Figure 2.5 shows typical blebs observed in the endothelial mosaic of an eye wearing a 38%-water-content HEMA lens with thickness of 0.15 mm (the lens producing the lowest PO_2 on the cornea in earlier PO_2 studies; see Figure 2.3). The response was similar for a 38%-water-content HEMA lens with a thickness of 0.09 mm. In contrast,

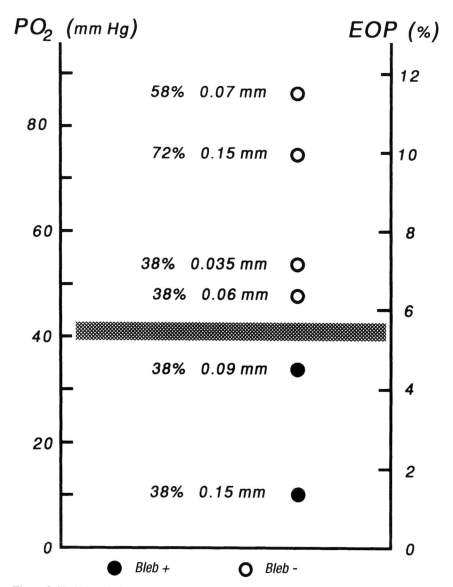

Figure 2.6 Relationship between oxygen tension (PO_2) under the contact lens and bleb formation with the eyelids open. Equivalent oxygen pressures (EOP) were calculated from PO_2. (Reprinted with permission from H Hamano. Overview of contact lenses in regard to corneal complications. J Jpn Contact Lens Soc 1995;37:1.)

thinner (0.06 and 0.035 mm) HEMA lenses and lenses with higher water contents (58% and 72%) produced no blebs. With the eyelids closed, however, all of these lenses induced bleb formation in the endothelial mosaic after 20 minutes. In the absence of a lens, absolutely no bleb formation was noted.

Figures 2.6 and 2.7 combine the results of the bleb formation studies with PO_2s measured under these lenses with the eyelids open (see Figure 2.6) and with the eyelids closed (see Figure 2.7). On the basis of these figures, it appears that the threshold for bleb formation is a PO_2 of approximately 40–45 mm Hg. When the PO_2 on the epithelial surface is higher than this, hypoxic effects (i.e., blebs) do not appear in the endothelium.

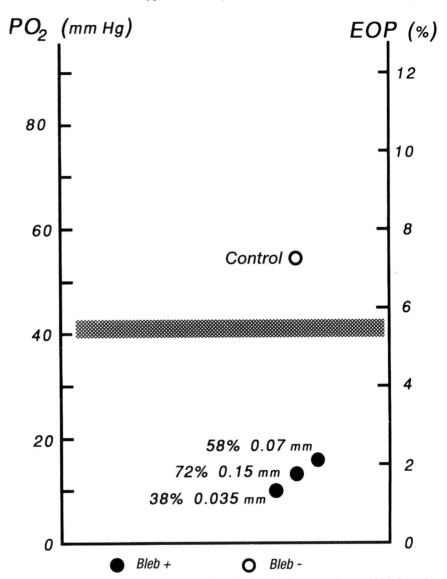

Figure 2.7 Relationship between oxygen tension (PO_2) under the contact lens and bleb formation with the eyelids closed. Equivalent oxygen pressures (EOP) were calculated from PO_2. (Reprinted with permission from H Hamano. Overview of contact lenses in regard to corneal complications. J Jpn Contact Lens Soc 1995;37:1.)

At present, however, there are no soft lenses that can maintain such high levels of oxygen with the eyelids closed. Thus, it could be that physiologic changes occur in the cornea when lenses are worn overnight, no matter how high the oxygen permeability of the lens.

OVERNIGHT CORNEAL SWELLING

Corneal swelling with overnight lens wear and the resultant deswelling have been studied by many investigators. The guidelines proposed by Holden and Mertz (1984)

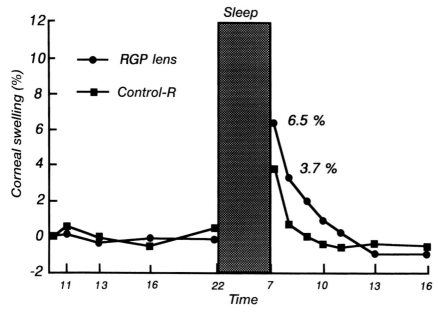

Figure 2.8 Corneal swelling and deswelling in an eye wearing a rigid gas-permeable (RGP) lens (Menicon Super EX) for 30 hours, including overnight during sleep. Control values (Control-R) were obtained in the same eye without a lens at least 1 week prior to the test measurements. Time on the x axis is given in clock hours (i.e., from approximately 10 A.M. one day until 4 P.M. the following day. (Reprinted with permission from R Sakamoto, Y Miyanaga, H Hamano. Soft and RGP lens corneal swelling and deswelling with overnight wear. Int Contact Lens Clin 1991;18:214.)

for "zero residual swelling" have become a time-tested standard by which clinical feasibility for extended wear can be judged. A number of the studies done in this area have concentrated on rates of deswelling (Andrasko 1986; Armitage and Schoessler 1988; Holden et al. 1988), but it is difficult to apply their results directly to the clinical situation.

In a study of overnight contact lens wear, Sakamoto et al. (1991) compared corneal swelling and deswelling for two types of extended-wear lenses: a high-Dk rigid gas-permeable lens (Dk = 216×10^{-11}, as reported by the Japanese manufacturer) and a soft disposable lens (50% water content, 0.07-mm thickness). Nine subjects with no contact lens experience participated in this study. A rigid gas-permeable lens was placed on the right eye, and a soft contact lens was placed on the left eye. The lenses were worn continuously for a period of 30 hours, including during sleep. Corneal thickness measurements were made at time 0 (10 A.M.) and 1, 3, 6, and 12 hours later on the first day, then at 7 A.M. (precisely at the time the eyes were opened in the morning) and 1, 2, 3, 4, 6, and 8 hours later on the second day. At least 1 week before the test measurements, control measurements were taken on the same schedule in both eyes with no lens wear.

Figures 2.8 and 2.9 show the time course of corneal swelling and deswelling for the rigid gas-permeable lens and the soft lens, respectively. With the rigid gas-permeable lens, overnight swelling was 6.5 ± 1.6% (see Figure 2.8). With the soft lens, overnight swelling was 10.0 ± 2.7% (see Figure 2.9); this is more than the 8% limit set by Holden and Mertz in 1984. Also, swelling with soft lens wear

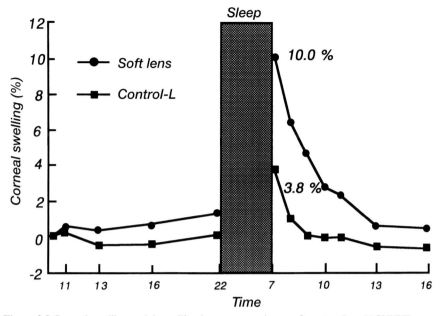

Figure 2.9 Corneal swelling and deswelling in an eye wearing a soft contact lens (ACUVUE, Johnson & Johnson, Jacksonville, FL) for 30 hours, including overnight during sleep. Control values (Control-L) were obtained in same eye without a lens at least 1 week before the test measurements. Time on the *x* axis is given in clock hours (i.e., from approximately 10 A.M. one day until 4 P.M. the following day). (Reprinted with permission from R Sakamoto, Y Miyanaga, H Hamano. Soft and RGP lens corneal swelling and deswelling with overnight wear. Int Contact Lens Clin 1991;18:214.)

was significantly greater ($p < .05$, *t*-test) than was swelling with rigid gas-permeable lens wear.

Recovery time was defined as the length of time after waking needed for the lens-wearing cornea to return to the thickness of the control eye. The rigid gas-permeable lenses allowed the cornea to deswell to the control level by 4 hours after waking. The corneas wearing soft lenses never returned to control level over the course of study (i.e., during a period of more than 9 hours after waking), however.

The results of these studies suggest that with the introduction of new contact lens materials with greater oxygen permeability (Dk) and oxygen transmissibility (Dk/L), overnight swelling and deswelling times will become important parameters by which to evaluate the performance of extended-wear lenses and their effect on the cornea.

REFERENCES

Andrasko GJ. Corneal deswelling response to hard and hydrogel extended wear lenses. Invest Ophthalmol Vis Sci 1986;27:20.

Armitage BS, Schoessler JP. Overnight corneal swelling response in adapted and unadapted extended wear patients. Am J Optom Physiol Opt 1988;65:155.

Barr JT, Schoessler JP. Corneal endothelial response to rigid contact lenses. Am J Optom Physiol Opt 1980;57:267.

Efron N, Holden BA. The corneal endothelium and conjunctiva. Contact Lens Monthly 1986;192:17.

Efron N, Kotow M, Martin DK, Holden BA. Physiological response of the contralateral cornea to monocular hydrogel contact lens wear. Am J Optom Physiol Opt 1984;61:517.

Hamano H, Hori M, Hamano T, et al. Effects of contact lens wear on mitosis of corneal epithelium and lactate content in aqueous humor of rabbit. Jpn J Ophthalmol 1983;27:451.

Hamano H, Mikami M, Mohri H, Mitsunaga S. Measurement of oxygen partial pressure at the rabbit cornea under various types of contact lenses [in Japanese]. J Jpn Contact Lens Soc 1984;26:295.

Hamano H, Mikami M, Mohri H, et al. Measurement of oxygen tension in anterior ocular segments by a platinum microelectrode: I. Preliminary experiments in vitro system [in Japanese]. J Jpn Contact Lens Soc 1986a;28:47.

Hamano H, Mikami M, Mohri H, et al. Measurement of oxygen tension in anterior ocular segments by a platinum microelectrode: II. In vivo measurement of oxygen tension on rabbit and human cornea under various gas-permeable hard contact lenses [in Japanese]. J Jpn Contact Lens Soc 1986b;28:51.

Hamano H, Watanabe K, Mitsunaga S. Observation of corneal endothelial response to hydrogel lenses by non-contact specular microscope (TOPCON SP1000) [in Japanese]. J Jpn Contact Lens Soc 1993;35:140.

Holden BA, Mertz GW. Critical oxygen levels to avoid corneal edema for daily and extended-wear contact lenses. Invest Ophthalmol Vis Sci 1984;25:1161.

Holden BA, Sweeney DF, Lahood D, Kenyon E. Corneal deswelling following overnight wear of rigid and hydrogel contact lenses. Curr Eye Res 1988;7:49.

Holden BA, Williams L, Zantos SG. The etiology of transient endothelial change in the human cornea. Invest Ophthalmol Vis Sci 1985;26:1354.

Sakamoto R, Miyanaga Y, Hamano H. Soft and RGP lens corneal swelling and deswelling with overnight wear. Int Contact Lens Clin 1991;18:214.

Schoessler JP, Woloschak MJ, Mauger TF. Transient endothelial changes produced by hydrophilic contact lenses. Am J Optom Physiol Opt 1982;59:764.

Vannas A, Holden BA, Makitie J. The ultrastructure of contact lens induced changes in the human corneal endothelium. Acta Ophthalmol (Copenh) 1984;62:320.

Williams L, Holden BA. The bleb response of the endothelium decreases with extended wear of contact lenses. Clin Exp Optom 1986;69:90.

Zantos SG, Holden BA. Transient endothelial changes soon after wearing soft contact lenses. Am J Optom Physiol Opt 1977;54:856.

3

The Tear Film and Contact Lens Wear

Takashi Hamano

Tears play an important role in successful contact lens wear. It is well known that tears of adequate volume and normal composition are required to ensure safety and comfort for wearers of contact lenses. Also well known is the fact that a high percentage of contact lens wearers with abnormally low levels of tear secretion have a variety of problems with lens wear, including staining, conjunctival hyperemia, superficial punctate keratopathy, corneal erosion, ocular discomfort, and foreign body sensation (Hamano et al. 1986). The relationship between contact lens wear and tears for the most part has not been elucidated fully thus far, however, partly because the tear film is changing constantly, owing to both environmental and physiologic factors. This chapter focuses primarily on the most recent theories concerning the relationship between contact lens wear and tears.

STRUCTURE OF THE TEAR FILM

Preocular Tear Film

Recently, the layer of tears that protects the exposed surface of the globe has come to be described as the *preocular* tear film rather than the *precorneal* tear film. This change is based on the recognition that both the cornea and conjunctiva are covered by the same tear film and that there is continuity between the two. Normal tears consist of a superficial lipid layer, a middle aqueous layer, and a mucin layer directly overlying the corneal or conjunctival epithelium.

In normal tears, the superficial lipid layer has a reticular pattern (Figure 3.1). This pattern is formed when lipids secreted from the meibomian glands spread thinly and widely over a mucin-coated surface (Hamano 1992) (Figures 3.2–3.4). If abnormally large amounts of lipids are secreted from the meibomian gland or if the tear turnover is poor, the lipid layer thickens, and a colorful interference pattern is seen on the surface (Figure 3.5). Most normal subjects display the reticular pattern; only approximately 5% of normal eyes exhibit the interference pattern. Approximately 25% of patients with dry eye exhibit the interference pattern, which also is seen more often in older patients than in younger patients, however.

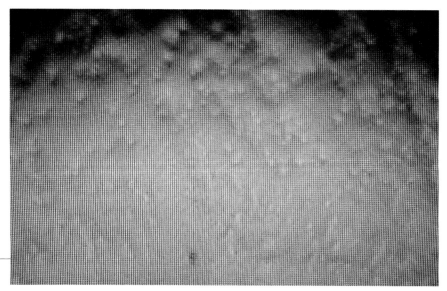

Figure 3.1 The superficial layer of the preocular tear film exhibiting a reticular pattern. Most normal eyes show this pattern. (Noncontact specular microscopy.)

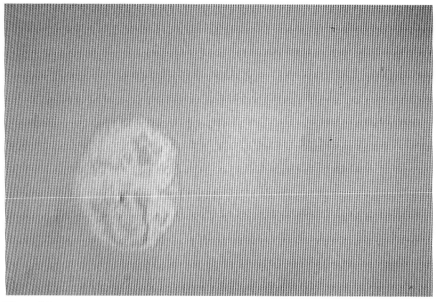

Figure 3.2 Two granules secreted from the meibomian gland. One already is beginning to spread to form the lipid layer of the tear film. (Noncontact specular microscopy.)

The normal reticular pattern of the superficial lipid layer indicates a normal lipid layer thickness of approximately 0.1 μm or less. The interference pattern, particularly one that displays multiple layers, indicates a lipid layer thickness of more than 1 μm. Because the interference pattern is seen more frequently among older patients and those with dry eyes, this pattern also may be a sign of reduced tear turnover.

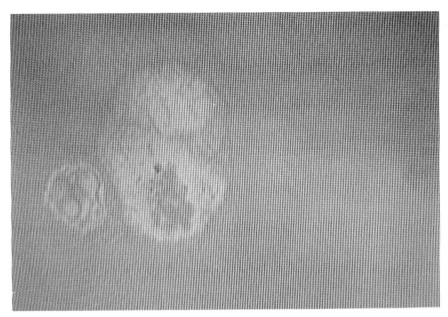

Figure 3.3 The second granule also beginning to spread, demonstrating the colors of an interference pattern. (Noncontact specular microscopy.)

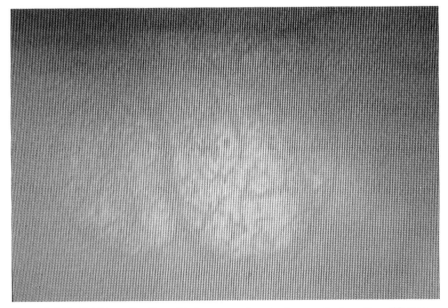

Figure 3.4 The lipid layer blending with the aqueous layer to form a reticular pattern. (Noncontact specular microscopy.)

In patients with severely dry eyes, especially those with Sjögren's syndrome, the lipids secreted from the meibomian glands sometimes do not spread out over the tear surface and instead form oil drops (Figure 3.6). This abnormality may be caused either by inhibition of lipid spread due to a reduction in the amount of mucin (Holly 1973) or by changes in the properties of the secreted lipids themselves. Observation

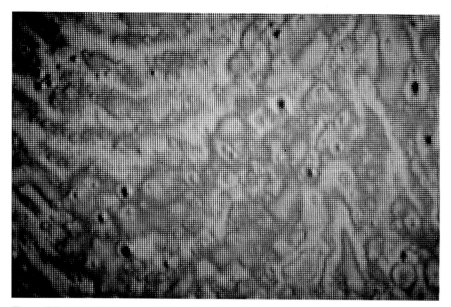

Figure 3.5 A thick lipid layer exhibiting the colors of an interference pattern. (Noncontact specular microscopy.)

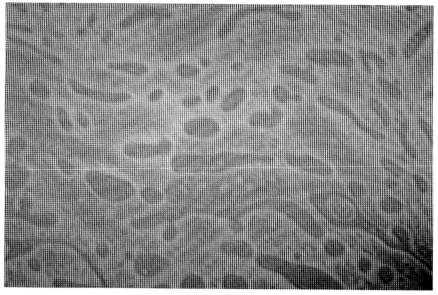

Figure 3.6 Secretions from the meibomian gland in a patient with Sjögren's syndrome. (Noncontact specular microscopy.)

of the tear film in both normal and dry eyes is facilitated with the use of a specially modified noncontact specular microscope (Hamano et al. 1990; Hamano 1991, 1992) or with the maximum magnification of a slit-lamp biomicroscope.

Our knowledge of the mucin layer has expanded significantly during the last decade. Until recently, our basic understanding has been that the corneal surface is primarily hydrophobic but becomes hydrophilic as the mucin secreted by the conjunctival goblet cells is spread over the corneal surface by blinking; this change makes it possible to maintain a stable tear film. Recent studies (Greiner et al. 1980, 1985; Dilly and Mackie, 1981; Dilly 1985; Gipson et al. 1992; Watanabe et al. 1995) have revealed, however, that the keratoconjunctival epithelial cells themselves secrete glycoprotein as well. No conclusion has been drawn yet concerning the relationship between the roles played by mucin originating from conjunctival goblet cells and by mucin originating from the keratoconjunctival epithelial cells. The general view is that, although the latter makes the ocular surface hydrophilic, the former dissolves in the aqueous layer to facilitate the spreading of the tears over the ocular surface.

Tear Film Breakup

In normal eyes, the preocular tear film covers the keratoconjunctival surface and is renewed with each blink. After each blink, most of the tear film begins to move superiorly as soon as the eyelids are opened; this shift is thought to be caused by the movement of the upper eyelid. Two or three seconds after the lids are opened, the tear film stabilizes, and movement stops. In normal eyes, the tear film remains stable for 10–20 seconds, with little or no breakup. When blinking is prevented and the eyelids are kept open continuously, the tear film gradually thins until it finally ruptures and exposes the epithelial cells (Figures 3.7 and 3.8).

Tear breakup time in normal eyes is relatively long, and the dry spots generally appear in only a few areas. In some people, the tear film shows no breakup at all for several minutes. In the dry-eye patient, however, the tear film breaks up quickly and in multiple areas (Figures 3.9–3.12). In severe cases, the tear film is completely absent in certain areas, exposing the cells (Figure 3.13). In such cases, the tear film often is already broken up immediately after blinking. Thus, these eyes remain continuously dry, which results in damage to the keratoconjunctival epithelium.

In general, when fluorescein sodium is instilled in the eye to measure tear breakup time, as is commonly done in the clinical setting, the recorded time to breakup is shorter than are the times observed with noninvasive forms of measurement (Mengher et al. 1985, 1986; Hamano et al. 1989; Hamano et al. 1989, 1993a).

TEAR FILM AND CONTACT LENS WEAR

Prelens Tear Film

The tear film on the surface of contact lenses is thin enough to exhibit the interference pattern; estimates of the thickness of the prelens tear film range from approximately 200 to 400 nm (Figure 3.14). Here, the interference pattern is generated not by the lipid layer but by the aqueous layer, which is extremely thin. Although the reticular pattern seen in normal eyes is also present in most cases, it is difficult to see because of the strong colors of the interference pattern.

The tear film that is spread over the surface of the contact lens by blinking recedes from the lens surface within several seconds after the eyelids are opened. The tears may recede in any direction, either superiorly, laterally, or uniformly

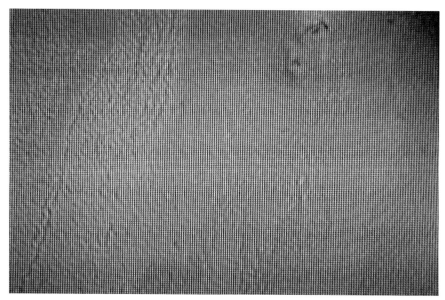

Figure 3.7 The tear film at the beginning of the tear breakup process. With blinking in normal eyes, this occurs approximately 10–20 seconds after the eyelids are opened. (Noncontact specular microscopy.)

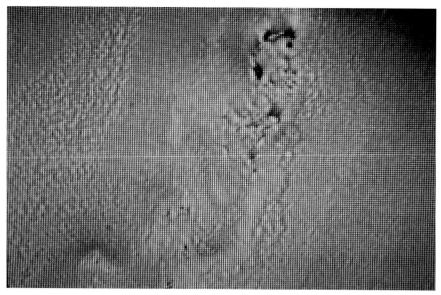

Figure 3.8 Expanded area of tear breakup with time. This expansion is limited in normal eyes. (Noncontact specular microscopy.)

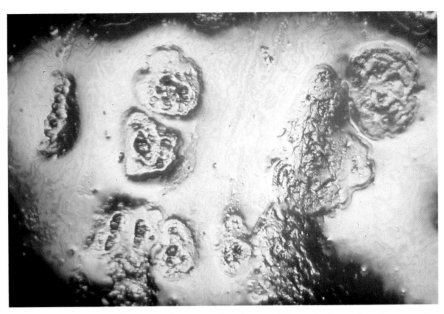

Figure 3.9 Tear film breakup over a larger area in a dry eye. (Noncontact specular microscopy.)

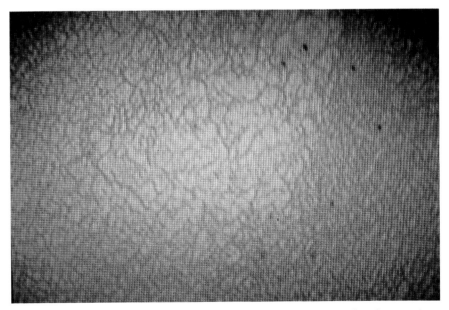

Figure 3.10 An example of multiple areas of tear breakup. (Noncontact specular microscopy.)

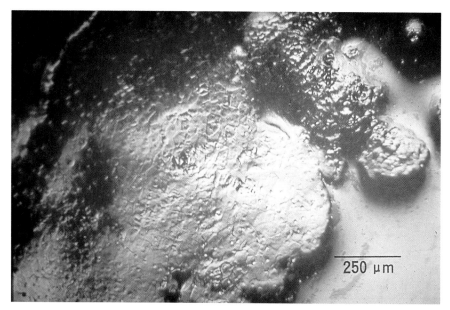

Figure 3.11 Corneal epithelial cells visible at the base of a dry spot. (Noncontact specular microscopy.)

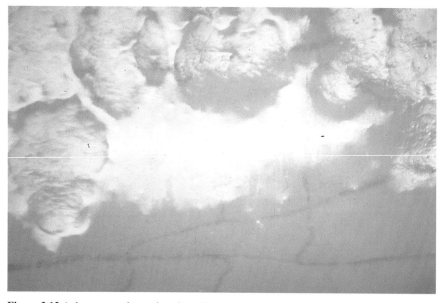

Figure 3.12 A dry spot on the conjunctiva. (Noncontact specular microscopy.)

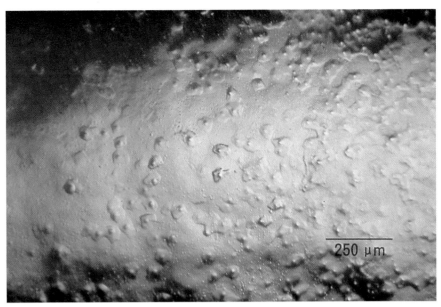

Figure 3.13 The corneal epithelium visible in an area close to the limbus with virtually no visible tear film. (Noncontact specular microscopy.)

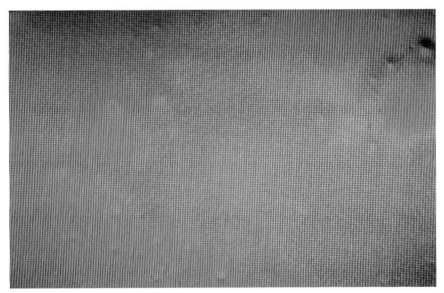

Figure 3.14 The prelens tear film on the surface of a rigid gas-permeable lens showing the colors of an interference pattern. (Noncontact specular microscopy.)

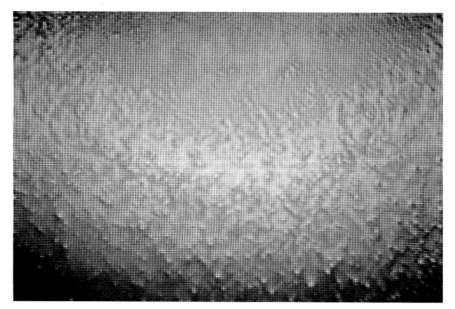

Figure 3.15 The prelens tear film on the surface of a rigid gas-permeable lens seen receding superiorly. (Noncontact specular microscopy.)

(Figures 3.15–3.17). The stability of the prelens tear film is determined by the condition of the contact lens surface. For the most part, the prelens tear film tends to be more stable when the contact lenses are new, probably because the surface of a contact lens becomes less hydrophilic with increasing wear. We found that the tear film receded from the surface of a new rigid gas-permeable lens in 6–7 seconds, but after the lens was worn for several months, the lens surface appeared dry within 2–3 seconds. Although there was some variation in the stability of the prelens tear film depending on the contact lens material, the differences were not significant.

Tear Volume and Contact Lenses

Patients with keratoconjunctival damage due to contact lens wear often have dry eyes. The incidence of keratoconjunctival damage has been reported to be roughly five times higher in patients with dry eyes than in normal patients (Hamano et al. 1986). In another study of patients with reduced tear secretion, those who wore hard contact lenses experienced significantly more pain, foreign body sensation, and hyperemia, and those who wore soft lenses experienced significantly more discomfort and dryness than did those patients with normal tear volumes (Hamano et al. 1989).

Tear Film Disruption in the 3 and 9 O'Clock Positions in Wearers of Rigid Gas-Permeable Lenses

Damage to the keratoconjunctival epithelium at the 3 and 9 o'clock positions, along with accompanying hyperemia, is common among wearers of rigid gas-

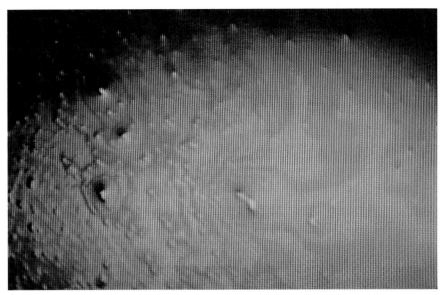

Figure 3.16 The prelens tear film on the surface of a rigid gas-permeable lens seen receding laterally. (Noncontact specular microscopy.)

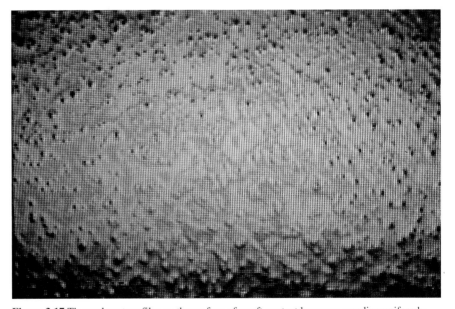

Figure 3.17 The prelens tear film on the surface of a soft contact lens seen receding uniformly. (Noncontact specular microscopy.)

permeable lenses. One study showed signs of this type of regional damage in roughly 40% of all hard contact lens wearers (Hamano et al. 1989). This problem occurs when the tear film in the 3 and 9 o'clock regions, which is unstable by nature, becomes more unstable, owing to increased dryness in these areas resulting from contact lens wear.

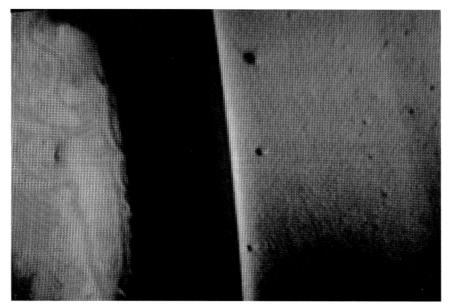

Figure 3.18 Tear film at 3 o'clock in a normal left eye wearing a rigid gas-permeable lens. (Non-contact specular microscopy.)

In patients with no damage to the keratoconjunctival epithelium in these regions, the tear film remains stable and is spread over the area with each blink (Figure 3.18). In patients with epithelial damage in the 3 and 9 o'clock positions, the tears are spread over the area immediately after blinking but dry up a few seconds later (Figure 3.19). With repeated blinking, the cycle of wetting and drying is thought to trigger the damage to the keratoconjunctival epithelium seen in these areas. This phenomenon may be considered a localized form of dry eyes because the changes closely resemble those of dry eyes (Figure 3.20).

Treatment of the keratoconjunctival epithelial damage is focused on preventing the localized dryness. In some cases, symptoms may be improved by changing the size and/or fit of the contact lens, which can alter the condition of the tear film. Instructing patients to consciously blink more often is also sometimes effective. Viscous eye drops can prevent local dryness to some extent. In a recent study, eye drops containing sodium hyaluronate were reported to decrease both the damage to the epithelium (Itoi et al. 1993) and the accompanying hyperemia (Hamano et al. 1993b).

Dryness in the Inferior Cornea in Wearers of Soft Contact Lenses

Wearers of soft contact lenses often complain of a feeling of dryness in their eyes. A number of studies have examined the relationship between soft contact lens wear and tear evaporation, but no clear conclusions have been reached. The symptom seen most frequently in wearers of soft contact lenses is superficial punctate keratopathy in the 6 o'clock area, which coincides more or less with the area where the initial damage to the corneal epithelium appears in patients with dry eyes. It has been suggested that this part of the eye is more susceptible to damage because the

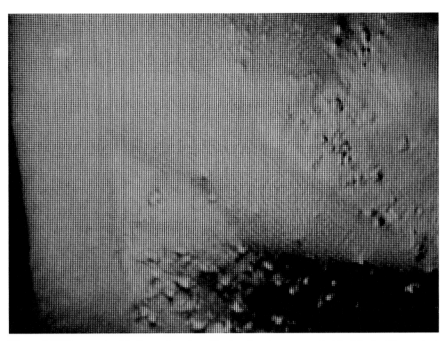

Figure 3.19 Damaged epithelium where tear film breakup has occurred at 3 o'clock. (Noncontact specular microscopy.)

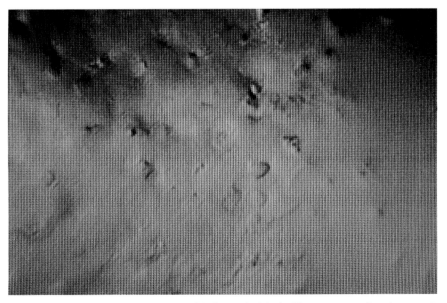

Figure 3.20 A dry eye showing damaged epithelium at 3 o'clock. (Noncontact specular microscopy.)

surface of the contact lens in this area is exposed for extended periods. That is, wearers of soft contact lenses often do not close their eyelids completely when they blink, permitting localized drying of the inferior portion of the lens surface (Watanabe et al. 1994).

Blinking and Contact Lenses

Compared with people who do not wear contact lenses, a large number of people who wear hard contact lenses blink in an incomplete manner. If the eyelids do not close completely during blinking, the tear film is not distributed normally, not only over the contact lens but also over the keratoconjunctiva in the adjacent 3 and 9 o'-clock areas. As a result, these areas dry out and remain dry.

Similarly, people engaged in work requiring high visual concentration, such as driving and computer operation, are known to blink less frequently, although not necessarily in an incomplete manner. Normally, people blink between 20 and 30 times a minute. However, those playing video games, for instance, blink much less often, sometimes as seldom as four to five times a minute or even as rarely as once every other minute. In this type of situation, even if the eyelids close completely with each blink, the cornea and conjunctiva easily become dry, and the result is damage to the keratoconjunctival epithelium in the 3 and 9 o'clock regions.

Thus, for contact lens wearers, blinking is most important because it significantly affects the disposition of the tears over the surface of the contact lens and the adjacent keratoconjunctival epithelium. Blinking also is essential for a smooth exchange of tears beneath the contact lens. Therefore, maintaining an adequate frequency of blinking and closing the eyelids completely with each blink are two very important factors in ensuring the safety and comfort of contact lens wearers.

REFERENCES

Dilly PN. On the nature and the role of the subsurface vesicles in the outer epithelial cells of the conjunctiva. Br J Ophthalmol 1985;69:477.

Dilly PN, Mackie IA. Surface changes in the anaesthetic conjunctiva in man, with special reference to the production of mucus from a non-goblet-cell source. Br J Ophthalmol 1981;65:833.

Gipson IK, Yankauckas M, Spurr-Michaud SJ, et al. Characteristics of a glycoprotein in the ocular surface glycocalyx. Invest Ophthalmol Vis Sci 1992;33:218.

Greiner JV, Kenyon KR, Henriques AS, et al. Mucus secretory vesicles in conjunctival epithelial cells of wearers of contact lenses. Arch Ophthalmol 1980;98:1843.

Greiner JV, Weidman TA, Korb DR, Allansmith MR. Histochemical analysis of secretory vesicles in nongoblet conjunctival epithelial cells. Acta Ophthalmol (Copenh) 1985;63:89.

Hamano H, Kotani S, Mitsunaga S, et al. Incidence of 3 and 9 o'clock staining caused by rigid contact lens wear [in Japanese]. J Jpn Contact Lens Soc 1989;31:253.

Hamano T. Pre-ocular tear film and the contact lens [in Japanese]. J Eye 1991;8:1707.

Hamano T. Specular microscopy of pre-ocular tear film [in Japanese]. J Eye 1992;9:1659.

Hamano T, Hamano T, Hamano H, et al. Contact lens wear troubles and phenol-red thread test [in Japanese]. J Jpn Contact Lens Soc 1986;28:104.

Hamano T, Horimoto K, Lee M, Komemushi S. Evaluation of the effect of the sodium hyaluronate ophthalmic solution on tear film stability—non-contact specular microscopic evaluation [in Japanese]. J Jpn Ophthalmol Soc 1993a;97:928.

Hamano T, Horimoto K, Lee M, Komemushi S. Evaluation of the effect of sodium hyaluronate ophthalmic solution on corneal desiccation due to hard contact lens wear [in Japanese]. J Eye 1993b;10:627.

Hamano T, Mitsunaga S, Kotani S, et al. Relationship between age, contact lens wear and tear volume [in Japanese]. J Jpn Contact Lens Soc 1989;31:68.

Hamano T, Watanabe M, Danjo Y. Non-contact specular microscopy for the ocular surface evaluation—non-invasive specular microscopy of the pre-ocular tear film and corneal epithelium of normal subjects and dry eye patients [in Japanese]. J Eye 1990;7:1190.

Holly FJ. Formation and rupture of the tear film. Exp Eye Res 1973;15:515.

Itoi M, Kim O, Kimura T, et al. The effect of sodium hyaluronate ophthalmic solution on corneal epithelial disorders in contact lens wearers [in Japanese]. J Eye 1993;10:617.

Mengher LS, Bron AJ, Tonge SR, Gilbert DJ. A non-invasive instrument for clinical assessment of the pre-corneal tear film stability. Curr Eye Res 1985;4:1.

Mengher LS, Pandher KS, Bron AJ, Davey CC. Effect of sodium hyaluronate (0.1%) on break-up time (NIBUT) in patients with dry eyes. Br J Ophthalmol 1986;70:442.

Watanabe H, Fabricant M, Tisdale AS, et al. Human corneal and conjunctival epithelia produce a mucin-like glycoprotein for the apical surface. Invest Ophthalmol Vis Sci 1995;36:337.

Watanabe K, Lee M, Hamano T, Tano Y. Analysis of blinking patterns and tear evaporation patterns in contact lens wear. J Jpn Contact Lens Soc 1994;36:179.

4

Corneal Topography*

Stephen D. Klyce and Naoyuki Maeda

The cornea produces approximately two-thirds of the refractive power of the human eye, in addition to its other functions, such as transparency and protection. The refractive power of the cornea is determined in large part by the anterior corneal curvature and its uniformity, and these factors have an important effect on the optical quality of the eye. Strictly speaking, the greatest refractive power of the human eye is located not at the tear-cornea interface but at the interface between the tear film and the air; for this reason, most current methods of corneal topographic analysis actually measure the surface of the tear film rather than the surface of the cornea itself. The term *corneal topography* is used, however, with the understanding that the surface under consideration is that of the cornea and the overlying tear film.

The evolution of keratorefractive surgery required new methods that can evaluate corneal shape more sensitively and accurately, and corneal topographic analysis was designed to provide the information needed by refractive surgeons to assess the results of their procedures. Today, the analysis of corneal shape within the entrance pupil is used for assessing the outcome of refractive surgery. Also, the analysis of central topography is important for assessing the effect of contact lenses on corneal optics. Additionally, analysis of the topography of the corneal periphery can provide important data for improving contact lens fitting. Thus, what was developed as a laboratory research tool beginning little more than a decade ago has, within the last 5 years, become a widely used, commercially available diagnostic instrument with a variety of applications in the clinical setting.

CORNEAL GEOGRAPHY

Anatomic Divisions of the Corneal Surface

For convenience in clinical discussion, the corneal surface can be divided anatomically into three zones. The central zone is defined as the area within a circle ap-

*This work was supported in part by United States Public Health Service grants EY03311 and EY02377 from the National Eye Institute, National Institutes of Health, Bethesda, MD, and by funds from Computed Anatomy, New York, NY, and from Menicon Co., Ltd., Nagoya, Japan.

proximately 4 mm in diameter, over which the cornea is thought to be relatively spherical (Waring 1989). Although there is no real consensus about the exact location of the central zone, this region is best defined in terms of the optical function of the cornea (i.e., the central zone can be designated as the corneal projection of the entrance pupil under daylight conditions). Thus, the central zone is the most important optical component of the cornea, through which high-resolution images are formed on the fovea.

The paracentral zone is an annulus that circumscribes the central zone. In this zone, the peripheral flattening of corneal curvature generally becomes more pronounced. The topography of the paracentral zone gains optical importance under dim illumination as the pupil enlarges. Also, precise information about the shape of the paracentral zone is useful in contact lens fitting.

The limbal zone includes the junction of the cornea and the sclera. The cornea is flattest in the limbal zone.

Geometric, Anatomic, and Optical Centering Points on the Cornea

The geometric center of the cornea can be located by estimating or by calculating the mathematic centroid of the limbal outline. It is used sometimes as a reference point for marking the resting position of the contact lens.

The center of the apparent entrance pupil is located by having the patient fixate properly on a point coincident with the line of sight of the observer (Uozato and Guyton 1987). This is the point that should be used for centering the optical zone of a contact lens and the optical zone for refractive surgical procedures.

The corneal vertex is the perpendicular intersection of the fixation light with the anterior corneal surface. It is important in corneal topography because all keratoscopic images are centered on this point. The corneal vertex does not always coincide with either the center of the entrance pupil or the geometric center of the cornea. Usually, it is slightly inferonasal to the center of the entrance pupil. Topographic analysis systems should provide data on the location of the pupil compared with that of the corneal vertex for use in refractive surgery and contact lens fitting.

METHODS OF TOPOGRAPHIC ANALYSIS

Keratometry

Keratometry, either manual or automated, is used to perform one of the most important clinical examinations for the prescription of contact lenses and the calculation of intraocular lens power. The manual keratometer projects one illuminated target ring onto the cornea from a fixed distance determined by focus and alignment. Measurements are taken at only four points 3–4 mm apart. The maximum and minimum diameters of the equivalent ellipse are determined, and the curvatures are obtained by comparison with the diameters measured on calibration spheres. Using these measurements, the radius of curvature of the central cornea and the amount and axis of astigmatism, if any, are calculated (Dabezies and Holladay 1986). The keratometry readings, or K readings, are the corneal refractive powers obtained by keratometry. Corneal refractive power (C_p, expressed in diopters) can be calculated directly from the radius of curvature (R_c, expressed in millimeters) using the following equation:

$$C_P = \frac{337.5}{R_c}$$

where 337.5 represents the keratometric index.

The automated keratometer projects mires onto the cornea with infrared light and detects their positions with infrared detectors, all within approximately 40 milliseconds. Thus, the readings are objective and require minimal intervention by the operator. An automated keratometer may have a video screen to simplify alignment and focusing. Maximum and minimum corneal curvatures and the axis of astigmatism are calculated automatically, and these data are displayed on the screen and are printed out. The information provided by the automated keratometer generally is more accurate and reproducible than are the readings obtained with the manual keratometer (Holladay and Waring 1992).

Although both manual and automated keratometers are reasonably accurate, reliable, and useful for measuring corneal contours, both have some noteworthy limitations. As mentioned earlier, they measure corneal curvature at only four points separated by 3–4 mm on the paracentral cornea. No data are obtained from the central cornea, although such data would be important for assessing the dioptric power of the central cornea for intraocular lens calculations, nor are data available from the peripheral cornea, the area on which contact lenses ride. Finally, the keratometry calculations are based on the assumption that the cornea is a spherocylindrical surface and asphericity or asymmetry of corneal shape cannot be detected. However, not only corneas with irregular astigmatism but also normal corneas may have topographies that deviate from the spherocylindrical (Dingeldein and Klyce 1989). Therefore, keratometry is not appropriate for the accurate evaluation of optical quality, contact lens fitting, or surgical results in corneas that differ noticeably from this ideal shape.

Photokeratoscopy

The photokeratoscope uses a Placido disk to project multiple concentric target rings on the cornea and records the resulting mire images photographically. In comparison with the keratometer, this instrument can obtain topographic information from a larger part of the corneal surface because of the additional rings.

Qualitative analysis of keratoscope photographs can provide significant information (Rowsey et al. 1981). Abnormalities of the corneal contours are identified by the systematic visual inspection of the keratoscope mire patterns (Figure 4.1). Examples of keratoscope photographs are shown in Figure 4.2 (normal cornea), Figure 4.3 (moderately advanced keratoconus), and Figure 4.4 (contact lens–induced warpage). Although the visual inspection of mire patterns has the advantage of relatively low cost and speed in the detection of obvious corneal distortions, corneal shape anomalies that have significant impact on vision often cannot be detected with this method. Even for the experienced user of photokeratoscopy, regular astigmatism of less than 3 diopters (D) or mild changes in corneal asphericity cannot be appreciated by visual inspection of mire patterns.

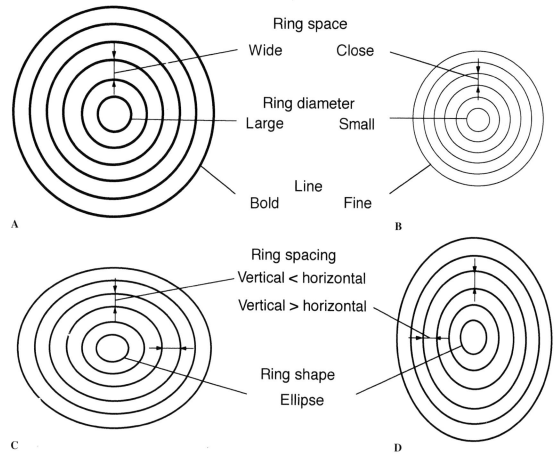

Figure 4.1 Visual inspection of the mire pattern. A. Flat. B. Steep. C. With-the-rule astigmatism. D. Against-the-rule astigmatism. The diameter, spacing, and width of the reflected mires are influenced by corneal power. Small-diameter, closely spaced, and narrow rings are seen in steep regions (elevated surface power or shorter-than-usual radius of curvature). Elliptical distortion of mires is the hallmark of regular astigmatism, with the long axis of the ellipse falling on the flattest (lowest-power) meridian. Irregular spacing between rings and ring tortuosity are characteristics of irregular astigmatism.

Videokeratography

The videokeratoscope is a keratoscope that uses a video camera to capture the image of the mires. Then, computer digitization of the video image allows the automatic reconstruction of corneal shape. Since the late 1980s, a variety of videokeratography instruments have become available commercially. All project concentric circular rings onto the cornea and digitize their locations automatically. Each instrument, however, has different features involving the details of the Placido disk, focusing methods, reconstruction algorithms of the corneal shape, and presentation schemes.

One instrument, the TMS-1 (Computed Anatomy, New York, NY), has a 25- or 30-ring collimating photokeratoscope cone. Refractive power information can be obtained from as many as 6,400 to nearly 8,000 data points (Gormley et al. 1988). In this system, the distance between each mire is approximately 0.17 mm on the corneal surface, and the inner ring leaves only a 0.45-mm diameter area of central cornea unexamined.

Figure 4.2 Keratoscope photograph of a normal cornea. The circular shape of the central rings, their concentric nature, and their width produce uniform spacing along every meridian. These are the characteristics of mire patterns in a cornea with a uniform power distribution and with no marked evidence of astigmatism.

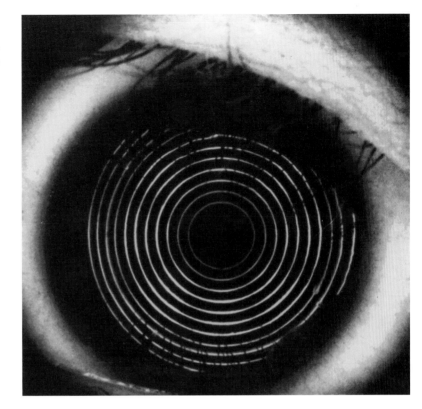

Figure 4.3 Keratoscope photograph of a cornea with moderately advanced keratoconus. The diameters of the central rings are smaller than normal, indicating a high surface power. The mires are not concentric, and the width of the rings is not uniform. The rings become quite narrow, especially in the interior paracentral regions of the cornea, indicating an area of steepening.

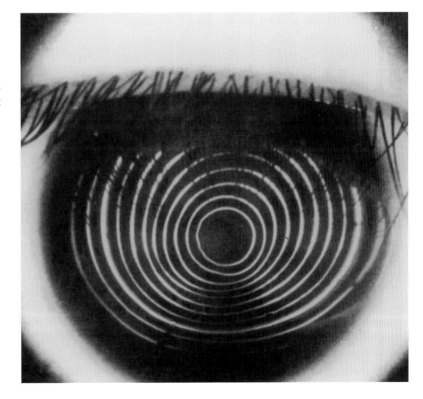

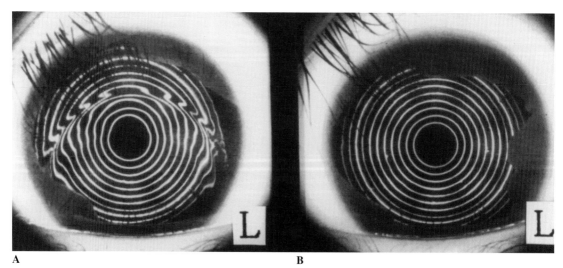

A   B

Figure 4.4 Keratoscope photographs of a cornea (A) with contact lens–induced corneal warpage and (B) after a period with no contact lens wear. The contact lens was a rigid gas-permeable lens that was decentered inferiorly in the resting position. The distortion of the cornea includes an arcuate-shaped irregularity of the mires along the lens margin and irregularities in the central rings (A). After lens wear was discontinued for 1 month, the cornea resumed its normal shape (B).

With the use of a cone that fits inside the orbital ridge, data from the limbal zone can be obtained without shadows created by the ridge of the brow or by the nose. The 25-ring cone provides data from an area of the cornea approximately 9 mm in diameter; the 30-ring cone, which was designed primarily for contact lens work, provides information from an area almost 10.5 mm in diameter (Klyce and Dingeldein 1990).

The Color-Coded Dioptric Contour Map

In videokeratography, the color-coded map is used to display corneal surface power distribution. The idea behind these maps is to present useful topographic information in a manner that permits speedy interpretation of corneal contour through pattern recognition coupled with identification of normal-abnormal corneal powers specified by a predefined, color-coded scale (Maguire et al. 1987). In the color scale, greens and yellows are used to code corneal dioptric powers that generally are representative of powers found in the central zone of the normal cornea. Cool colors (violets, blues) symbolize lower than normal corneal powers, and warm colors (oranges, reds) indicate higher than normal corneal powers. The Klyce-Wilson scale uses 26 intervals with 1.5-D steps, ranging from 28.0 to 65.5 D. This range, which is almost identical to that measured by manual and automated keratometers, provides the best combination of sensitivity for detection of clinically significant topographic features and coverage of the wide range of powers that may be found in a cornea after refractive surgery (Wilson et al. 1993).

Another approach to color coding of topographic maps is the normalized scale, or adaptive color scale (Gormley et al. 1988), which expands or contracts its range to fit the range of powers present in a given topographic map. This method is able to show great topographic detail, but its disadvantage is that the reproducible color associations as described earlier are lost, precluding easy visual comparisons from map to map. Also, with this approach, normal corneas sometimes can be made to look quite abnormal, and truly abnormal corneas can be made to appear closer to normal (Figures 4.5 and 4.6).

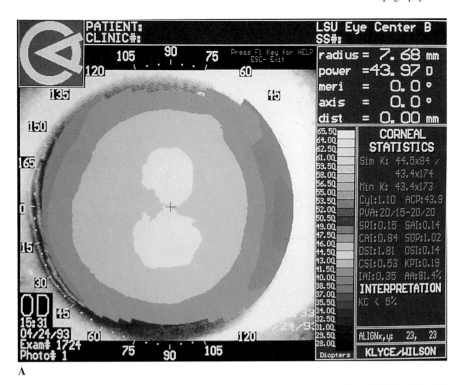

A

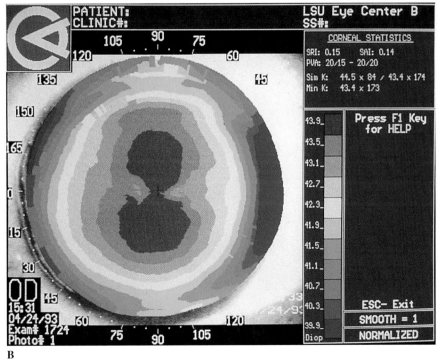

B

Figure 4.5 Comparison of the topographic appearance of a normal cornea by using (A) the Klyce-Wilson scale and (B) the normalized scale. Note that a relatively small amount of astigmatism is exaggerated by the normalized scale.

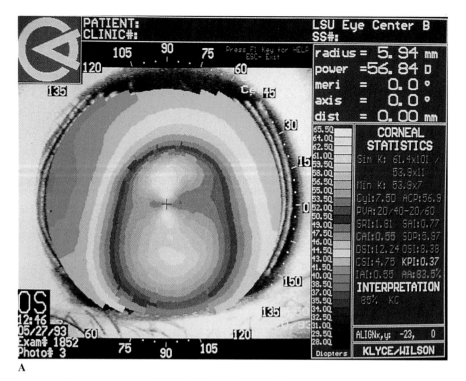

A

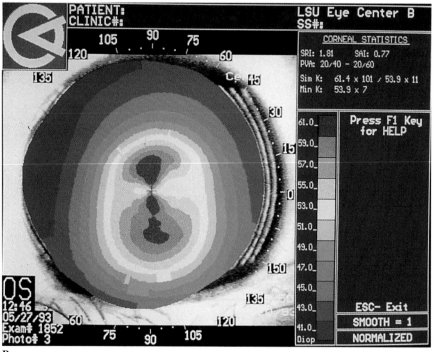

B

Figure 4.6 Comparison of the topographic appearance of a cornea with keratoconus by using (A) the Klyce-Wilson scale and (B) the normalized scale. With the normalized scale, the color-coded map resembles the appearance of with-the-rule astigmatism.

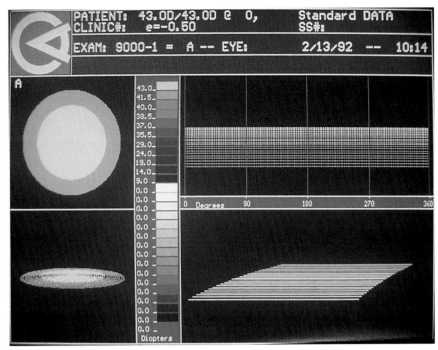

Figure 4.7 Schematic drawing of an isometric graph of a normal cornea. The lines are horizontal and parallel to each other, indicating that this cornea has peripheral flattening and no astigmatism.

The Isometric Graph

Raw data obtained with the videokeratoscope can be shown as a two-dimensional graph that plots values in diopters along the vertical (y) axis, and degrees along the horizontal (x) axis for all rings (Hamano et al. 1990). This graph is called an *isometric graph* because corneal refractive powers are plotted isometrically for any angle. A completely spherical cornea would be shown as a series of straight lines parallel to the horizontal axis (Figure 4.7). Regular astigmatism would be displayed as a sine curve that has two phases over 360 degrees (Figure 4.8). Asphericity is represented by an increase or decrease in the height of the curves for peripheral rings as compared to those of central rings. The isometric graph is particularly sensitive in the detection of localized irregular astigmatism along each ring and the detection of abnormal asphericity along semimeridians.

Quantitative Analysis of the Topographic Map

Although a considerable amount of qualitative information is provided by the color-coded map through pattern recognition and color association, this type of evaluation is not useful for the analysis of the results of a clinical trial involving multiple visits by a large group of patients at multiple centers. For this purpose, numeric indices that could be subjected to statistical testing were developed by derivation from the raw topographic data. These indices are useful both for comparisons among patients and groups and for following individual patients longitudinally to guide therapy and to assess its effects.

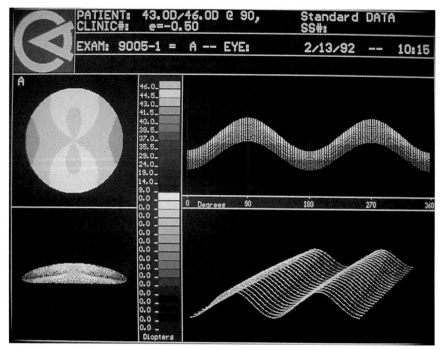

Figure 4.8 Schematic drawing of an isometric graph of a cornea having with-the-rule astigmatism. The smooth sine curve displays the regularity of the astigmatism, and the uniform widths of the curves indicate that the degree of asphericity is the same in every semimeridian.

Some of the quantitative indices that have been developed for the TMS-1 videokeratoscope are shown in Table 4.1. The simulated keratometry reading (SimK) correlates well with the values obtained from separate keratometry measurements (Dingeldein et al. 1989). The surface asymmetry index (SAI) is a centrally weighted summation of differences in corneal power between corresponding points 180 degrees apart on 128 equally spaced meridians crossing all mires (Dingeldein et al. 1989). Theoretically, the SAI value would be zero for a perfect sphere, for a surface with perfectly spherocylindrical regular astigmatism, and for any surface with a power that is radially symmetric. Thus, the higher the SAI, the more asymmetric the corneal surface.

The surface regularity index (SRI) indicates local power fluctuations along each of the 10 central mires (Klyce et al. 1989). The SRI correlates with localized surface regularity within the central area of the cornea corresponding approximately to the area of the entrance pupil. A high correlation between the SRI and best spectacle-corrected visual acuity was shown in a prospective study (Wilson and Klyce 1991). Therefore, the SRI can be used to predict the potential visual acuity of a given patient with an otherwise normal eye, on the basis of the surface quality of the central cornea.

Other characteristics of corneal topography can be analyzed by developing quantitative indices that are sensitive to certain features in the topographic maps. With experience, the examiner can learn to interpret topographic abnormalities based on these indices and to understand the relationship between the topographic map appearance and specific features of the corneal power distribution.

These indices also are being used to develop automated keratoconus detection schemes based on various types of artificial intelligence methodology, including ex-

Table 4.1 Quantitative Indices Produced by TMS-1 Topographic Analysis

Index	Parameter Measured
SimK (simulated keratometry)	Simulated value of keratometry readings
MinK (minimum keratometry)	Power and axis of the actual flattest meridian
SAI (surface asymmetry index)	The extent of radial symmetry in the measured cornea
SRI (surface regularity index)	Refractive power fluctuation in the central cornea
IAI (irregular astigmatism index)	Refractive power fluctuation in the measured cornea
AA (analyzed area)	Ratio of the interpolated area to the measured area
CAI (corneal asphericity index)	Asphericity in the central cornea
SDP (standard deviation of power)	Refractive power variation in the measured cornea
I-S (inferior-superior value)	Refractive power difference between inferior and superior paracentral cornea

pert classifier systems and neural networks (Rabinowitz and McDonnell 1989; Klyce et al. 1994; Maeda et al. 1994). In the future, the clinician may be able to obtain a preliminary indication of the cause of corneal shape anomalies through automated interpretation of the topographic pattern or through quantification of specific topographic features, as a guide and support for the results of clinical evaluation and diagnostic judgment.

CLINICAL APPLICATIONS OF VIDEOKERATOGRAPHY

Normal Cornea

Understanding the topographic characteristics of the normal cornea helps in the interpretation of color-coded maps of both normal and abnormal corneas. Among the common characteristics of the topography of the normal cornea (Figure 4.9) is a gradual flattening of approximately 2–4 D from the center to the periphery (Dingeldein and Klyce 1989). The nasal semimeridians generally are more flattened than are the temporal semimeridians. Spherical aberration in the eye probably is corrected to some extent by this aspherical feature. Normal corneas exhibit a degree of smoothness, or absence of significant irregular astigmatism. The appearance of irregular astigmatism in the normal cornea frequently reflects the presence of dry eyes, contact lens wear, or a history of ocular surgery.

Corneas display topographic pattern variations that usually are unique to the individual, much like fingerprints, allowing identification. Topographic maps of the two corneas from one individual normally exhibit nonsuperimposable mirror-image symmetry (enantiomorphism); this feature can be helpful in the differential diagnosis of unilateral diseases.

Astigmatism

Regular astigmatism is the most common naturally occurring topographic pattern seen in the optically adequate normal cornea (Figure 4.10). In most cases, regular corneal astigmatism is with-the-rule, with the steep axis at 90 degrees, but oblique and against-the-rule corneal cylinders also are found in regular corneal astigmatism.

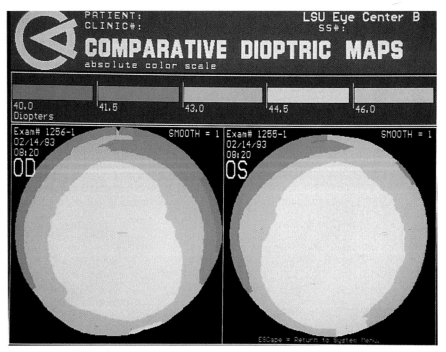

Figure 4.9 Color-coded maps of the left and right eyes of an individual with normal corneas. Both corneas have a smooth and homogeneous dioptric power distribution in the center, with radial symmetry and progressive peripheral flattening. The maps display nonsuperimposable mirror images (enantiomorphism) to the medial line.

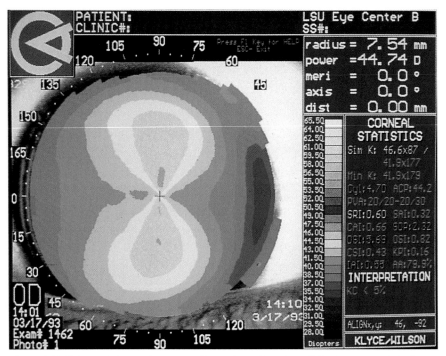

Figure 4.10 Color-coded map of a cornea with regular astigmatism. This shape anomaly is displayed as a vertically aligned bow-tie pattern with elevated corneal power. The superior and inferior portions are symmetric to the flattest axis of the astigmatism.

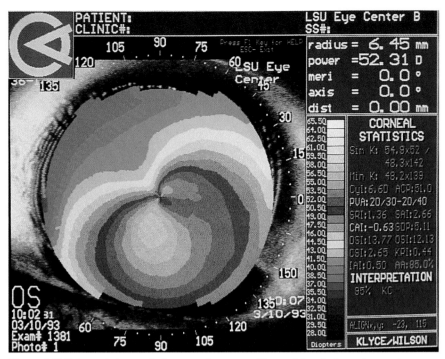

Figure 4.11 Color-coded map of a keratoconic cornea with a peripherally located cone. An area of localized steepening is found in the inferior cornea. The color-coded map also shows obvious asymmetry and a large difference in power between the steepest and flattest areas.

The topographic appearance of regular astigmatism is displayed in the color-coded map as a bow-tie–shaped pattern with radial symmetry. For example, simple with-the-rule astigmatism produces a vertically aligned bow-tie pattern of higher corneal surface power.

All corneal topographic deviation from a purely ellipsoidal shape generally is considered to be irregular astigmatism. Irregular astigmatism has various causes, such as keratoconus, contact lens–induced warpage, ocular surgery, and trauma and is displayed in a variety of patterns with topographic analysis. When irregular astigmatism occurs within the pupillary area or when a highly aspherical surface is present, vision may be impaired.

Keratoconus

The characteristic topographic findings of the keratoconus patient include high central corneal power, a cornea with an inferior region steeper than the superior region, a large difference between the corneal power of the apex and that of the periphery, and a disparity in the central corneal power between the two eyes of a single patient (Rabinowitz and McDonnell 1989). Approximately 75% of keratoconus patients have peripheral cones with steepening extending to the limbus (Figure 4.11), and these cones typically are restricted to one or two quadrants (Wilson et al. 1991). Approximately 25% of keratoconus patients have central corneal steepening (Figure 4.12). Occasionally, the apex of the cone is located in the superior quadrant (Wilson et al. 1991).

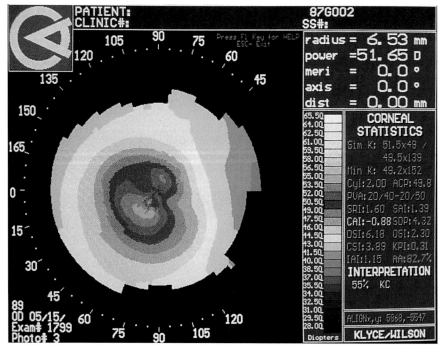

Figure 4.12 Color-coded map of a keratoconic cornea with a centrally located cone. This map has abnormal steepening in the center. Note that the bow-tie pattern is shifted 90 degrees to form a "lazy eight" pattern.

Because keratoconus patients do not achieve good vision with spectacles, owing to irregular astigmatism, they tend to select either contact lens wear or refractive surgery for optical correction (Wilson and Klyce 1994). Refractive surgery is likely to produce unstable or otherwise unsatisfactory results in eyes with keratoconus, however, and therefore the diagnosis of this disorder is an essential part of the presurgical evaluation. Videokeratography offers virtually the only clinical approach to the diagnosis of early keratoconus (Maguire and Bourne 1989) (Figure 4.13). Using the Klyce-Wilson scale, videokeratographs of keratoconus-suspect corneas are characterized by a local area of corneal steepening, generally located in an inferior quadrant. The eyes of patients who fall into the category of keratoconus-suspect must be followed with serial topographic analysis to determine whether the condition progresses to clinically diagnosable keratoconus.

Contact Lens Wear

Contact Lens–Induced Corneal Warpage

Contact lens–induced corneal warpage can be found in wearers of both soft and rigid contact lenses. The topographic alterations found in color-coded maps of corneas with this type of warpage consist of central irregular astigmatism, loss of radial symmetry, and frequent reversal of normal progressive flattening from the center to the periphery (Wilson et al. 1990a, 1990b) (Figure 4.14). Usually a loss of radial symmetry in the topographic map is associated with the resting position of the contact lens, and flat-

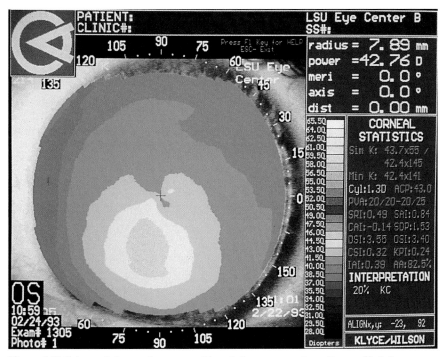

Figure 4.13 Color-coded map of a cornea with early keratoconus. A small area of inferior steepening is seen. Note that the simulated keratometry (SimK) value (42.7/43.7 × 55) is within the normal range (41–45).

tening occurs at the paracentral corneal area under the decentered lens. This finding suggests that a rigid contact lens should be fitted to maintain a well-centered resting position. Although corneal warpage caused by soft contact lens wear can reverse to the normal pattern with 4–6 weeks of cessation of lens wear, in most cases as much as 5 months may be required to restore and stabilize normal corneal topography after rigid lens wear is discontinued. Corneal power may be altered by as much as 1.0 D, either flatter or steeper, during this stabilization period. Occasionally, corneal topographic warpage becomes permanent, and significant irregular astigmatism, a permanent reduction in best-corrected spectacle visual acuity, or both can result.

Similar corneal topographic changes have been found even in visually normal eyes of patients who have worn either rigid or soft contact lenses with no symptoms (Ruiz-Montenegro et al. 1993). In this study, topographic changes tended to be more frequent and more severe in patients wearing rigid gas-permeable lenses than in patients wearing soft contact lenses. Similarly, SAI and SRI values were significantly higher in corneas that wore rigid contact lenses compared with normal control values. The majority of corneas in contact lens–wearing patients had values within the normal range, however.

Pseudokeratoconus and Contact Lens Wear

The topographic changes caused by a rigid contact lens with a superior resting position are similar to those seen in patients with early keratoconus; this form of contact lens–induced corneal warpage is termed *pseudokeratoconus*. The recommended method for

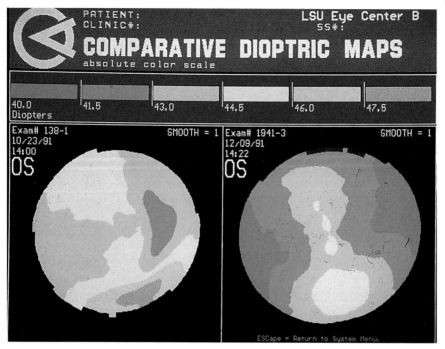

Figure 4.14 Sequential color-coded maps of a cornea with contact lens–induced warpage. Left. The rigid gas-permeable lens worn in this eye had a superior nasal resting position. The topographic map shows inferior steepening. Right. One month later. Although the topographic pattern displayed a more normal bow-tie pattern after a well-centered rigid gas-permeable lens was fitted, there is still a small asymmetry in the map.

differentiating contact lens–induced warpage from keratoconus is to discontinue contact lens wear until corneal topography is stabilized. If the "keratoconus pattern" stabilizes to a bow-tie pattern, it is likely that contact lens warpage was the cause of the topographic changes. If the keratoconus pattern persists, it may indicate either permanent warpage due to contact lens wear or keratoconus. If there are no other clinical signs of keratoconus, the patient should be advised to cease wearing contact lenses for at least 6 months, after which topographic analysis should be repeated. In patients who have worn contact lenses and are, in fact, developing true keratoconus, the keratoconus pattern sometimes becomes more prominent after lens wear is discontinued because certain types of cones tend to be flattened by contact lenses. If the patient cannot or will not abandon contact lens wear for this period, a lens that rides centrally in its resting position should be fitted; this will allow any contact lens–induced corneal warpage to diminish.

Another useful method to differentiate keratoconus from contact lens–induced warpage is comparison of the topographies of the patient's two eyes. Contact lens–induced pseudokeratoconus often produces similar patterns in both eyes, whereas true keratoconus frequently is more advanced in one eye than in the other.

Computer Simulation of the Fluorescein Pattern

Fitting rigid gas-permeable lenses sometimes can be a very time-consuming, trial-and-error process. This is particularly true of irregular astigmatism patients, for whom rigid lens wear usually is critical to obtaining good visual acuity.

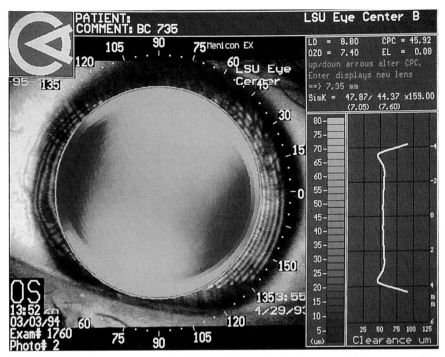

Figure 4.15 Computer simulation of the fluorescein examination in an eye with keratoconus. The correspondence between the real pattern and the simulation is excellent, even when the cornea has irregular astigmatism, such as keratoconus. The clearance between the contact lens and the cornea in all meridians is shown in the line plot on the right.

Because corneal topographic analysis involves the reconstruction of the corneal surface, the data also can be used to create a simulation of a fluorescein test in an eye with a particular rigid gas-permeable lens prescription (Figure 4.15). The effects of back-surface optical zone diameters, peripheral curves in the multicurve-design lens, or asphericity changes in the aspherical-design lens on the fluorescein pattern can be assessed before a special custom-made lens is ordered. It is also possible to estimate the changes in the fluorescein pattern caused by the decentration of the resting position of the lens (Klyce et al. 1992).

Topographic Analysis of the Contact Lens Surface In Situ

Soft contact lenses usually have low material rigidities and flex to conform to the anterior corneal contour. Therefore, they can undergo in situ flexure, which affects their design parameters. Topographic analysis of the soft contact lens in situ can be useful to evaluate the effects of such changes on the optical quality of the lens when it is in place on the eye. In one study (McCarey et al. 1993), the effects of toric soft contact lenses on corneal astigmatism were examined topographically. These authors found that spherical soft contact lenses failed to mask corneal astigmatism and even produced an increase in some cases. Toric soft contact lenses were able to neutralize corneal astigmatism to some extent, however.

The surface topography of contact lenses that had been worn for some period was compared with that of new, replacement lenses in the same eyes (Hamano et al.

1992). Irregular topographic patterns were seen in the color-coded maps of the worn soft contact lenses but were not seen in the maps of the new soft lenses, even though the new lenses had the same parameters as did the worn lenses. Additionally, the SRI and SAI of the worn lenses were significantly higher than were the values for the new lenses.

CONCLUSION

Corneal topography analysis is becoming an essential and routine clinical tool for the ophthalmologist, providing a variety of capabilities that include the diagnosis of corneal shape disorders, diagnosis of the underlying causes of irregular astigmatism, and diagnosis of the effects of irregular astigmatism on the optical performance of the eye, and serving as a guide to the fitting of contact lenses.

REFERENCES

Dabezies OH, Holladay JT. Measurement of Corneal Curvature: Keratometer (Ophthalmometer). In OH Dabezies (ed), Contact Lenses: The CLAO Guide to Basic Science and Clinical Practice, Vol. 1. Orlando, FL: Grune & Stratton, 1986;17.

Dingeldein SA, Klyce SD. The topography of normal corneas. Arch Ophthalmol 1989;107:512.

Dingeldein SA, Klyce SD, Wilson SE. Quantitative descriptors of corneal shape derived from computer-assisted analysis of photokeratographs. Refract Corneal Surg 1989;5:372.

Gormley DJ, Gersten M, Koplin RS, Lubkin V. Corneal modeling. Cornea 1988;7:30.

Hamano H, Hamano T, Hamano T, et al. Comparison between old and new soft contact lenses' surface shape during wear. J Jpn Contact Lens Soc 1992;34:53.

Hamano H, Sawa M, Maeda N, et al. Fundamental and clinical studies of corneal physiology and contact lenses (part 1). Asia-Pac J Ophthalmol 1990;2:42.

Holladay JT, Waring GO. Optics and Topography of Radial Keratotomy. In GO Waring (ed), Refractive Keratotomy for Myopia and Astigmatism. St. Louis: Mosby, 1992;37.

Klyce SD, Dingeldein SA. Corneal Topography. In B Masters (ed), Noninvasive Diagnostic Techniques in Ophthalmology. New York: Springer, 1990;61.

Klyce SD, Estopinal HA, Gersten M, et al. Fluorescein exam simulation for contact lens fitting [ARVO abstract]. Invest Ophthalmol Vis Sci 1992;33(suppl):697.

Klyce SD, Maeda N, Smolek MK. Use of neural networks for interpretation of corneal topography: I. Initial demonstration [ARVO abstract]. Invest Ophthalmol Vis Sci 1994;34(suppl):2079.

Klyce SD, Wilson SE, Pittman SD, Wang J. Estimation of potential visual acuity from corneal shape [ARVO abstract]. Invest Ophthalmol Vis Sci 1989;30(suppl):218.

Maeda N, Klyce SD, Smolek MK, Thompson HW. Automated keratoconus screening with corneal topography analysis. Invest Ophthalmol Vis Sci 1994;35:2749.

Maguire LJ, Bourne WM. Corneal topography of early keratoconus. Am J Ophthalmol 1989;108:107.

Maguire LJ, Singer DE, Klyce SD. Graphic presentation of computer-analyzed keratoscope photographs. Arch Ophthalmol 1987;105:223.

McCarey BE, Amos CF, Taub LR. Surface topography of soft contact lens for neutralizing corneal astigmatism. CLAO J 1993;19:114.

Rabinowitz YS, McDonnell PJ. Computer-assisted corneal topography in keratoconus. Refract Corneal Surg 1989;5:400.

Rowsey JJ, Reynolds AE, Brown R. Corneal topography. Corneascope. Arch Ophthalmol 1981;99:1093.

Ruiz-Montenegro J, Mafra CH, Wilson SE, et al. Corneal topography alterations in normal contact lens wearers. Ophthalmology 1993;100:128.

Uozato H, Guyton DL. Centering corneal surgical procedures. Am J Ophthalmol 1987;103:264.

Waring GO. Making sense of keratospeak: II. Proposed conventional terminology for corneal topography. Refract Corneal Surg 1989;5:362.

Wilson SE, Klyce SD. Quantitative descriptors of corneal topography: a clinical study. Arch Ophthalmol 1991;109:349.

Wilson SE, Klyce SD. Screening for corneal topographic abnormalities before refractive surgery. Ophthalmology 1994;101:147.

Wilson SE, Klyce SD, Husseini ZM. Standardized color-coded maps for corneal topography. Ophthalmology 1993;100:1723.

Wilson SE, Lin DTC, Klyce SD, et al. Topographic changes in contact lens–induced corneal warpage. Ophthalmology 1990a;97:734.

Wilson SE, Lin DTC, Klyce SD, et al. Rigid contact lens decentration: a risk factor for corneal warpage. CLAO J 1990b;16:177.

Wilson SE, Lin DTC, Klyce SD. Corneal topography of keratoconus. Cornea 1991;10:2.

II

Contact Lenses

5

Development of Contact Lenses

George W. Mertz

In contrast to *history*, which is an account of all that has happened, *development* relates more to stages of growth or advancement (McKechnie 1983). Most of the history of contact lenses is trial and error, with far more failures than successes. Still, successes have occurred, and today's contact lenses, although not perfect, have never been better and have never been worn by more patients worldwide. Technology has been the primary driving force behind the development of modern contact lenses.

Contact lens history has been studied with much greater authority and detail than is intended here (Mandell 1988; Heitz 1989; Sabell 1989). In this chapter, the development of contact lenses is traced from the conception of the idea of a contact lens to the most recent advancement in the contact lens field and the subject of this book, disposable contact lenses. From a historical perspective, only successes that have had a direct impact on the development of modern contact lenses, particularly disposable contact lenses, are included.

EARLY DEVELOPMENT OF CONTACT LENSES

The Idea of a Contact Lens

Mandell (1988) defines a contact lens as

> a small, shell-shaped device of plastic or similar material in the form of a lens that is in contact with the cornea or sclera, or both, and which serves as a new anterior surface of the eye … [and] is self-supporting and remains in contact with the eye either by fluid attraction forces and/or the lids.

Leonardo Da Vinci often is credited with conceiving of the idea of a contact lens in his drawings, circa 1508. Whether his work can be interpreted as actually describing a true contact lens remains in dispute in the literature (Hofstetter and Graham 1953; Hofstetter 1984; Heitz 1989). The identity of the true first conceiver may be lost in history; however, the first written description of a contact lens probably can be attributed to an English astronomer, Sir John F. W. Herschel, who, in 1823, proposed the use of a glass shell filled with animal jelly to be worn on the eye in cases of irregular corneal astigmatism (Herschel 1845).

Invention of the First Contact Lens

The literature (Mandell 1988; Heitz 1989; Sabell 1989) is in agreement that the principle of a contact lens was first reduced to practice for visual improvement in the
late 1880s,* more or less simultaneously by three independent inventors: A. Eugen
Fick, an ophthalmologist from Zurich, Switzerland; Eugene Kalt, an ophthalmologist
from Paris, France; and August Müller, a medical student from Gladbach, Germany.

Fick (1888) published his clinical experience with contact lenses under the title *Eine
Contactbrille (A Contact Spectacle)*. His objective was to produce a regular anterior
surface on a distorted cornea. According to Mandell (1988), his initial device, tried first
on rabbit eyes, was a glass corneal lens with parallel front and back surfaces. Fick also
described using glass scleral lenses, which Mandell presumed he preferred because the
scleral flange provided better support and weight distribution of the heavy glass lens
than was possible with a corneal design. Others contend that Fick's contact lenses were
never corneal, but rather scleral in design from the beginning (Efron and Pearson 1988).

Also in 1888, a Professor Photimos Panas delivered to the French Academy of
Medicine in Paris a lecture in which he described the work of his junior colleague,
Eugene Kalt. Kalt devised glass corneal lenses, which he called *glass contact shells*,
for the treatment of keratoconus. The lenses are thought to have been cut from blown
glass bubbles (Heitz 1989).

Although Fick and Kalt developed contact lenses for corneal surface irregularities,
August Müller's efforts were directed at correcting his own refractive error (–14.00
diopters). He used glass lenses designed with a posterior curvature similar to the front
surface of the cornea and with an anterior surface of curvature necessary to correct the
refractive error. In his inaugural thesis at the University of Kiel (Müller 1889), Müller
described his experiences with his invention, which he called *hornhautlinsen*, or
corneal lenses. He was the first to use this now well-known term (Sabell 1989), although his lenses actually were corneoscleral in design (Mandell 1988; Heitz 1989).

DEVELOPMENT OF MODERN CONTACT LENSES

For at least four (and arguably as many as six) decades after the invention of contact
lenses in the late 1880s, very little occurred that might be considered relevant to the development of the contact lenses of today. (For details concerning this period, see the
excellent history references mentioned earlier: Mandell 1988; Heitz 1989; Sabell
1989.)

In this chronicle of the events leading to the development of the current generation of contact lenses, which covers the period from the 1930s to the present, three
general categories are considered: (1) the development of contact lens materials;
(2) the development of contact lens designs; and (3) the development of contact
lens manufacturing. A time line showing the developmental milestones for each
category is provided in Appendix 5.1.

---

*Centennial celebrations of the birth of the contact lens were held in 1987, prompted by the well-docu-
mented fabrication of the so-called Wiesbaden lens 100 years earlier (Bailey et al. 1987; Sabell 1989).
This contact lens was constructed by F. A. Müller, a maker of prosthetic eyes in Wiesbaden, Germany, at
the request of a physician, Dr. Theodore Saemisch, for a monocular patient whose remaining sighted eye
lacked normal eyelid function and needed protection from exposure to prevent total blindness. Therefore, the Wiesbaden lens holds the distinction of being the first therapeutic, or *bandage*, contact lens, but
it was not the first to be used as an aid to vision per se.

Development of Contact Lens Materials

Glass

All early contact lenses were made of glass. This is, of course, perfectly logical, because glass was perhaps the only transparent solid substance known at the time. The use of glass spectacle lenses to correct refractive errors was well understood. Glass was used commonly for ocular prostheses, so it was a natural extension to use glass to make the first contact lenses. Unfortunately, despite its outstanding optical characteristics, glass is impermeable to oxygen, and its high specific gravity makes it too heavy to permit the use of corneal designs for better tear exchange. Patients could tolerate wearing glass contact lenses only briefly before developing signs and symptoms of what we now know to be corneal oxygen deprivation (hypoxia). For these reasons, glass contact lenses met with very limited success (or, as some might argue, no success) throughout the entire period of their use.

Rigid Plastic

A major step forward occurred with the development of plastics in the 1920s and 1930s. In 1936, Dr. William Feinbloom invented a contact lens with an opaque plastic (resin) scleral flange portion and a central optical portion made of glass. This lens is regarded as the first effective use of plastic* in the fabrication of a contact lens (Feinbloom 1937; Knoll 1977).

Polymethyl methacrylate (PMMA) was invented in 1934 (Heitz 1989) and introduced in the United States by the Rhom and Haas Company in 1936 (Mandell 1988). PMMA, better known by its trade names Perspex, Plexiglas, and Lucite (Refojo 1994), soon was adopted as the contact lens material of choice, a distinction it was to hold for the next 35 or so years.

Theodore Obrig, a New York City optician, generally is credited with producing the first commercially viable PMMA lenses in 1939, but the literature is not entirely conclusive on this matter. Obrig apparently collaborated with Ernest Mullen, an engineer who succeeded in developing the PMMA molding process that Obrig used to produce the posterior surfaces of his PMMA lenses from molds made from colloidal impressions of his patients' eyes. A Hungarian ophthalmologist, Itsvan Gyorrfy, may deserve credit for the first PMMA contact lens, however. In a paper presented to the Hungarian Ophthalmological Society in 1939, he reported clinical results for patients whom he claimed to have fitted with PMMA lenses in 1938 (Bailey et al. 1987).

PMMA is transparent and has a much lower specific gravity than glass. The lower specific gravity, plus properties that allowed contact lenses to be fabricated in much thinner designs, made PMMA lenses (known more commonly as *hard contact lenses* since the development of soft lenses) very popular among contact lens fitters worldwide, primarily because of reduced weight and the resulting improvement in patient comfort (Mandell 1988).

---

*The first recorded attempt to use plastic as a contact lens material occurred in the late 1920s by the German company, Carl Zeiss (Knoll 1979). Zeiss owned the rights to German, British, and U.S. patents granted in 1922–1923 to a physics professor at the University of Halle, Albert Wigand, for contact lenses fabricated from cellon (cellulose acetate). Clinical trials sponsored by Zeiss failed due to polymer instability and ocular irritation.

PMMA offered a number of other advantages, including ease of fabrication (the material properties of PMMA being outstanding for lathing, polishing, cast molding, and even injection molding); suitability for in-office polishing and modification of parameters; outstanding optics; good surface wettability on the eye; strength and durability; parameter stability; and later, in corneal designs, rapid recovery from deformation (ability to correct corneal astigmatism effectively). In fact, were it not for one key problem—oxygen impermeability—the material properties of PMMA are such that it probably would be regarded as the most ideal contact lens material discovered to date.

Unfortunately, the oxygen impermeability of PMMA sealed its fate and thus its potential never could be fully realized. Eventually, it was recognized that the corneal oxygen deprivation occurring with PMMA lens wear was responsible for clinically observed physiologic problems related to hypoxia. It was obvious for many years that a contact lens material with all the positive attributes of PMMA plus oxygen permeability would be highly desirable. The search for such a material was the driving force behind the development of rigid gas-permeable (RGP) contact lenses.

The first RGP material to be approved by the United States Food and Drug Administration (FDA) was cellulose acetate butyrate in 1978 (Danker's Meso lens); however, this material never was well accepted because of stability problems. The first commercially successful RGP lens to be developed was the Polycon lens. The Polycon lens was a major breakthrough in rigid lens technology because its oxygen permeability often made the difference between failure and success for PMMA patients experiencing chronic hypoxia problems. It was made of a siloxane-methacrylate polymer invented in 1970 by Norman Gaylord, a polymer chemist, in collaboration with Dr. Leonard Seidner, a New York City optometrist and co-owner (with his brother) of Guaranteed Contact Lenses, a small contact lens manufacturing laboratory. They formed a company called Polymer Optics, Inc., which owned the Polycon lens and the U.S. patent covering the polymer issued to Gaylord in 1974. The company was sold to Syntex Ophthalmics in 1977, and the Polycon lens was released to the market in the United States shortly after FDA approval in early 1979 (Bailey et al. 1987; Barr and Bailey 1993; Refojo 1994).

Other RGP lens materials have been developed since, including silicone resins, fluoro-siloxane-methacrylates, and alkyl styrene copolymers. None of these RGP polymers, however, can be thought of as PMMA with oxygen permeability. The organic chemistry manipulations that lead to improvements in one material property (e.g., oxygen permeability) often compromise another property, such as wettability (Refojo 1994). In recent years, RGP materials developed with spectacular oxygen transmission properties have virtually eliminated the problem of corneal hypoxia, including during overnight wear. Even so, they are not entirely trouble free and, in some cases, are responsible for one or more of the following problems: poor wettability, attraction of surface deposits, adherence to the cornea, parameter instability, and slow recovery from deformation. Initial discomfort, however, is the primary reason for the failure of these improved RGP lenses to achieve greater acceptance by the contact lens–wearing population.

If one compares the clinical performance of RGP contact lenses with soft contact lenses in terms of vision, comfort, physiologic response, handling, and durability, RGP lenses generally outperform soft lenses in every category except one: initial comfort. Ironically, initial comfort is the one attribute that drives patient preference, particularly in the United States, where soft lenses have dominated the market during the last 15 years. RGP lenses are well accepted in some countries (e.g., Germany), where they account for more than 50% of the market. In the United States, however, they have never achieved more than a 15–20% share.

Soft Plastic

By a wide margin, soft contact lenses are the most successful class of contact lenses developed to date. Known also as *hydrophilic* or *hydrogel* contact lenses, they account for more than 80% of the worldwide contact lens market (Sulaiman and Holden 1993). The original hydrogel contact lens material, hydroxyethyl methacrylate (HEMA), was invented in 1954 by Professor Otto Wichterle and Dr. Drahoslav Lim of the Institute of Macromolecular Chemistry of the Czechoslovak Academy of Sciences in Prague. The discovery was an unexpected outcome of a comprehensive effort to find an ideal synthetic biomedical material for use in body implants (Wichterle 1978). The Czechs had outlined the basic requirements for such an ideal material. Two of those requirements were absence of extractable impurities and high permeability to water-soluble nutrients and metabolites. These requirements led Wichterle and his associates to pursue water-absorbing polymers (Wichterle 1978). One of their discoveries was the transparent gel material HEMA, which, when cross-linked for three-dimensional strength, was suitable for use in medical devices, including contact lenses. They received United States patents covering the invention in 1962 and 1965 (Refojo 1978).

Although Czech-produced HEMA lenses were distributed commercially in limited numbers in Western Europe under the trade name Spofalens beginning in 1962 (Dreifus 1978; Heitz 1989), it was only after a license for the North American and South American rights to the technology was purchased jointly in 1965 by Dr. Robert Morrison, an optometrist from Harrisburg, PA, and the National Patent Development Corporation (NPDC) of New York City that the stage was set for the unprecedented commercial success ultimately achieved by soft contact lenses. Shortly thereafter, the NPDC bought out Dr. Morrison's 50% interest and started searching for a partner with whom to commercialize the soft lens technology (Bailey et al. 1987). They approached most of the major hard contact lens manufacturers in the United States but encountered only skepticism and indifference. Eventually they turned to Bausch & Lomb of Rochester, NY, a leading manufacturer of precision instrumentation, ophthalmic equipment, and glass spectacle lenses.

At the time, Bausch & Lomb was facing severe financial hardship as a result of declining demand for its products, archaic manufacturing technology, and the growing popularity of plastic spectacle lenses versus glass. When a sublicensing agreement was reached and signed in 1966, it would prove to be the company's financial salvation, but not immediately. The company first had to undertake the formidable task of developing soft contact lens products for the U.S. market from the crude spin-casting machines provided by the Czechs. Then, just as the first product was nearing completion in 1968, the FDA suddenly classified the soft contact lens as a drug (Bailey et al. 1987), obligating the company to meet substantial additional regulatory requirements before the product could be released to the U.S. market.* There was speculation at the time that the government's action was influenced to some degree by the intense lobbying efforts of the hard contact lens industry, which had become intimidated by the prospect of competition from soft lenses (Bailey et al. 1987).

Bausch & Lomb finally received FDA approval in March 1971 and shortly thereafter introduced its Soflens (polymacon) contact lens, the first soft contact lens entry

---

*Since the passage of the Medical Devices Act of 1976, soft contact lenses have been classified as medical devices by the FDA.

to the world's largest marketplace. Only licensed eye care professionals with the legal right to prescribe or dispense contact lenses were allowed to purchase the lenses. Ironically, the FDA hurdle that Bausch & Lomb finally cleared (and the hard lens companies favored and possibly helped to create) now stood between those companies and any opportunity that they might have to share in the spectacular growth that was about to occur in the newly created soft contact lens market. For some, it would be a struggle for survival because with the success of soft lenses during the 1970s came the obsolescence of PMMA lenses. For Bausch & Lomb, it meant that the financial troubles of the past would soon turn to fortune because the company was about to enjoy a 3-year monopoly before its first competitor finally reached the U.S. market.

Although the soft contact lenses of the early and mid-1970s were tolerated by more patients and for longer periods of wear than previous lenses, they were far from trouble free. Many exaggerated claims were made about the capabilities of soft lenses, and misunderstandings about them were common. For instance, the early soft contact lenses were touted as capable of transmitting virtually all of the oxygen available from the atmosphere. Through the efforts of Professor Irving Fatt (University of California) and others, it soon was learned that the oxygen transmissibility of hydrogel lenses is proportional to polymer water content and the reciprocal of lens thickness (Fatt 1989). Some of the unexpected clinical problems encountered with the early lenses included corneal hypoxia, arcuate corneal staining, toxic responses to lens care solutions, inflammatory problems related to lens spoilation* and, occasionally, corneal infections.

The contact lens field owes a debt of gratitude to the researchers and clinicians whose dedication to scientific truth led to a much better understanding of the capabilities and limitations of contact lenses. Their efforts have been responsible for making modern contact lenses safer and more effective than they might otherwise be for millions of today's patients. A few are deserving of special mention, owing to the importance of their contributions to the body of knowledge about how the eye is affected by contact lens wear. In addition to the aforementioned Professor Fatt, the others include the team of Drs. Morton Sarver, Kenneth Polse, and Michael Harris of the University of California, for studies of the clinical and physiologic responses to contact lens wear; Boston optometrist Dr. Donald Korb, whose astute clinical observations and insights have been immensely valuable to the understanding of contact lens behavior; Dean Emeritus Richard Hill of Ohio State University, for studies of corneal response to alterations of environment induced by contact lenses and contact lens solutions; Dr. Hikaru Hamano and his colleagues of Osaka University in Japan, for their landmark research into how contact lens wear affects the corneal epithelium; Professor Montague Ruben of Moorfields Eye Hospital, London, for his work in the areas of contact lens–induced pathology and therapeutic applications of contact lenses; and Dr. Mathea Allansmith, for her pioneering research into the ocular immunologic response to contact lens wear, particularly contact lens–induced papillary conjunctivitis.

---

*Contact lens spoilation (Tripathi et al. 1978; Tighe 1989), or spoilage (Tripathi and Tripathi 1989; Hart 1993), is the surface buildup over time of (1) denatured proteins, lipids, inorganic precipitates, and other substances from the tears; (2) environmental pollutants, dust, pollen, and other airborne particles; (3) preservatives and other substances in contact lens care and maintenance products; and/or (4) microbes and microbial by-products.

Perhaps the most prolific and respected research center engaged in the study of contact lenses is the Cornea and Contact Lens Research Unit (CCLRU) located at the University of New South Wales in Sydney, Australia. The CCLRU was founded in 1976 by Professor Brien Holden, who is still its director. The thrust of the efforts of Holden and his team has been fourfold: (1) to understand the cornea better by studying how it responds to contact lens wear; (2) to generate the knowledge necessary to understand all aspects of contact lens behavior, particularly how lens wear affects all ocular tissues; (3) to propose and test strategies for improvements in contact lens performance; and (4) to evaluate the safety of products and to determine how well they achieve their intended purpose(s). (For a better understanding of contact lens performance criteria, based on nearly 20 years of CCLRU experience, see the CCLRU's published standards for successful contact lens wear [Terry et al. 1993].)

Improvements in soft contact lens performance occurred during the late 1970s and early 1980s with the development of thinner and larger lens designs and less toxic cleaning-disinfecting solutions. During the same period, there was a proliferation of soft contact lens products. Most of the lenses were made of copolymers of HEMA and one or more additional constituents. Such copolymers were developed either to provide different material properties (e.g., higher water content for greater oxygen permeability) or to circumvent the Czech patents, a strategy that was proved unsound when the NPDC won a patent-infringement suit on the matter in 1982 (Anonymous 1982).

The initial soft contact lenses introduced in the United States in the 1970s were low-water-content hydrogels (less than 50% water) and were approved by the FDA for daily wear only. In the late 1970s, a desire began to grow among U.S. consumers for lenses that could be worn for prolonged periods, including overnight during sleep. According to Zantos (1993), the development of such prolonged-wear lenses occurred in two phases: the European phase and the North American phase.

The European phase began in 1970 with the development of so-called continuous-wear or permanent-wear soft contact lenses, first pioneered by John de Carle, an English optometrist. de Carle reasoned that hydrogel lenses could be worn more or less continuously if the water content was increased substantially, thereby increasing oxygen transmission through the lens, and if the lens diameter was reduced to a size smaller than that of the cornea, thereby reducing inflammatory problems by reducing stimulation of the limbal vasculature (de Carle 1978). His lens, known by the trade name *Permalens* (perfilcon A), is a copolymer of HEMA, vinyl pyrrolidone, and methacrylic acid (Refojo 1994), with a water content of 71% (compared with 38.6% water for Wichterle's original HEMA material). Interest in continuous-wear lenses declined in Europe in the late 1970s, owing to reports of adverse responses and other clinical problems related primarily to lens spoilation and corneal hypoxia.

The North American phase followed soon thereafter. Just as interest in overnight wear was waning in Europe, it began increasing in the United States, driven by strong consumer demand for the convenience and freedom offered by overnight wear.* The terms *continuous wear* and *permanent wear* were discouraged by the

---

*In a survey published by Remba (1982), consumers were asked why they were interested in extended-wear lenses. Enhanced lifestyle freedom, such as taking a business trip or spending an evening away from home without the worries of lens care, topped the list. Also rated highly were the prospect of comfort improvement and the convenience associated with reduced care and handling. The ability to see on awakening was not rated as highly as the other reasons. This was viewed as a surprising result because anecdotally it was a commonly held belief among contact lens practitioners that the primary attribute driving their patients' strong demand for extended wear was their desire to see the clock dial during the night.

FDA, which favored the term *extended wear* to indicate that such lenses should be removed at finite intervals for routine cleaning and disinfecting. The FDA initially established radical guidelines for premarket approval of extended-wear lenses, including documentation of corneal thickness changes (pachymetry), corneal sensitivity (esthesiometry), and endothelial morphology (specular microscopy). This action drew strong criticism from the academic community as impractical (as only a few research centers had the equipment necessary to conduct the studies), prohibitively expensive, and nearly impossible to standardize (Fatt 1977; Kelly 1977). The guidelines soon were abandoned in favor of clinical studies that were similar to, although larger and longer than, those conducted for previous premarket approvals of new contact lens products.

de Carle sold the rights to manufacture and market the Permalens to a British company, Global Vision (UK) Ltd. of Southampton, England (Hodd 1977). The lens was introduced to the U.K. market in 1975. Global Vision soon was acquired by CooperVision of Sunnyvale, CA (now of Fairport, NY), which brought the lens to the United States. CooperVision sought FDA premarket approval for an extended-wear indication, which was granted in 1981. Approval also was given at that time for the Hydrocurve (bufilcon A) contact lens, which now is owned by Wesley-Jessen Corporation of Chicago, IL. These two lenses were the first extended-wear products approved by the FDA for cosmetic (nonaphakic) correction of simple refractive myopia. At the time, approval was granted for up to 30 days of extended wear before removal for cleaning and disinfecting.

It always was understood that extended-wear lenses would have to transmit more oxygen to the cornea than did daily-wear lenses because the source of oxygen to the cornea during closed-eye periods—the palpebral conjunctival blood vessels—provides only approximately one-third as much oxygen as does the atmosphere, the source during open-eye conditions. The oxygen transmissibility (Dk/L)* of a hydrogel contact lens can be increased either by increasing the water content of the polymer or by decreasing the thickness of the lens or by some combination of the two (Fatt 1989). With the approval of the Bausch & Lomb (polymacon) O3 and O4 series contact lenses for nonaphakic extended wear in 1983, the pattern was set for the three general strategies for optimizing the Dk/L of extended wear lenses: (1) high-water-content lenses, such as the Permalens, which had to be made relatively thick, owing to polymer fragility; (2) low-water-content lenses, such as the Soflens O3/O4 series, which were made very thin; and (3) medium-water-content lenses, such as the Hydrocurve, which could be made thinner than the high-water-content lenses and thicker than the low-water-content lenses.

A number of additional extended-wear products were approved by the FDA during the early to mid-1980s, and the market for these products grew rapidly. Despite very positive early anecdotal reports about extended wear (McEachern et al. 1982; Poster 1982), however, disenchantment steadily escalated as the number of

---

*As explained by Fatt (1989), the oxygen transmissibility of a contact lens is the amount of oxygen (per unit area per unit time) that passes through a contact lens to the cornea from its oxygen source. The oxygen transmissibility, or Dk/L, is defined as the oxygen permeability of the lens material, or Dk, divided by the thickness of the lens, L. Dk is the ability of oxygen to move through the material. For hydrogel lenses, the mechanism of oxygen passage is diffusion through the water in the material. The higher the water content of a material, the greater its Dk value. Therefore, if two hydrogel lenses are identical in design but made of two different polymers, the higher-water-content lens will have the greater oxygen transmissibility. Similarly, if two hydrogel lenses are made of the same polymer but are different in design, the thinner lens will have the greater oxygen transmissibility.

extended-wear patients experiencing clinical problems increased, apparently from the long-term effects of chronic corneal hypoxia and lens spoilation (Grant et al. 1990). These clinical problems included chronic and acute inflammatory responses (contact lens–induced papillary conjunctivitis, contact lens–related acute red eye) and ulcerative keratitis (sterile peripheral ulcers, microbial ulcers).

As a result of the circulating anecdotal reports about adverse responses associated with extended-wear lenses, an epidemiologic study was commissioned by the Contact Lens Institute, an industry trade association, to determine the incidence and relative risks of ulcerative keratitis associated with contact lens wear (Poggio et al. 1989; Schein et al. 1989). The study showed that the risk of ulcerative keratitis with soft contact lens wear was 5–15 times greater for extended wear than for daily wear and that the risk increased with the number of nights of extended wear. Based on these results, the FDA issued an extended-wear alert to practitioners and "suggested" to manufacturers that extended wear be limited to no more than 7 days and 6 nights of continuous wear without removal for cleaning and disinfection.

Disposable Contact Lenses

At the time of this writing, no important additional advancements in polymer development have been made beyond what has been described. Therefore, it follows that disposable contact lenses were developed by using conventional hydrogel materials. In fact, an argument can be made that this failure to develop improved polymers is precisely the reason for the development of disposable lenses.

Development of Contact Lens Designs

The two primary types of contact lens design are corneal and scleral (Mandell 1988). Corneal lenses rest on the cornea and have an overall diameter equal to or less than the size of the cornea (within the limbus). Scleral lenses actually are corneoscleral (i.e., larger than the cornea), covering both the cornea and a portion of the sclera (outside the limbus).

Scleral Designs

Even if Fick's earliest efforts were with glass corneal lenses (Mandell 1988), which is now disputed (Efron and Pearson 1988), he quickly abandoned this approach in favor of glass scleral lenses (Fick 1888). Because glass is so heavy, scleral designs would have been more comfortable and more stable on the eye. Glass corneal lenses were tried from time to time in the years that followed but never with any success (Sabell 1989).

Even after the invention of PMMA, scleral designs continued to dominate the field. Because PMMA could be cast molded, techniques were developed for producing PMMA scleral lenses by casting in molds made from colloidal impressions of the anterior ocular surface. Attempts to improve clinical performance were made by manipulating lens design but always within the context of an overall scleral design (Sabell 1989). Unfortunately, the oxygen impermeability of PMMA and the sealing-off effect of scleral designs generally resulted in corneal oxygen deprivation, which severely limited the length of time most patients found tolerable for lens wear. This problem was never overcome with scleral PMMA designs.

Polymethyl Methacrylate Corneal Designs

The year 1948 generally is regarded as the beginning of the modern era of contact lenses. In February of that year, the patent application for the first PMMA corneal contact lens was filed by Kevin Touhy of Solex Laboratories in Los Angeles. The primary advantage offered by this revolutionary combination of lightweight plastic and a corneal design was the potential for increased tear exchange behind the lens as an avenue for increased corneal oxygenation during lens wear. The posterior surface of Touhy's lens was a monocurve design. This feature restricted tear exchange behind the lens unless the lens was fitted much flatter than the central corneal radius. Such fitting tended to cause lens edge standoff with resulting discomfort as well as corneal problems such as surface distortion and central abrasions (Mandell 1988).

The addition of posterior peripheral curves that were flatter than the central posterior lens surface is credited to George Butterfield. The adoption of this design modification greatly improved the comfort and physiologic tolerance of the PMMA lens. Further improvements were accomplished by reducing the diameter and thickness of the lens. This type of PMMA lens design dominated the contact lens field until the development of soft contact lenses (Mandell 1988).

Soft Lens Designs

As might be expected, the PMMA corneal design served as the initial model for early soft contact lenses, which originally were less than 10 mm in diameter (Heitz 1989). It soon became evident, however, that the PMMA design was not going to work for the much more flexible soft lens. Soft lenses smaller than the cornea would not center and were blinked off the cornea easily by the eyelids. Lenses larger than the cornea proved more successful. Such designs, although scleral by the definition given earlier in this chapter, are called *semiscleral* instead because the distance that they extend outside the cornea is so much less (0.5–1.5 mm) than that of typical scleral lenses. All soft contact lenses in use today are semiscleral in design.

The initial Bausch & Lomb Soflens (polymacon) contact lens, known as the *C series*, was 13.5 mm in diameter and had a monocurve posterior surface. This product enjoyed only limited success, mainly because it was very thick in lower minus powers, which substantially reduced wearing time owing to corneal hypoxia.

The Bausch & Lomb C series lens soon was followed by the F series and N series lenses, which were thinner and 12.5 mm in diameter. The F and N series also had a posterior peripheral bevel design that was thought to enhance tear exchange. Additional 12.5-mm lenses were released to the market later (B series and J series) and, although these lenses were very successful commercially, they often decentered excessively. Because they were small by today's standards, such decentration often led to edge impingement on the peripheral cornea on the side opposite to the direction of decentration. Clinicians discovered that lens edge impingement typically resulted in mechanical trauma to the cornea epithelium, a form of keratitis known as *arcuate corneal staining*, because of its characteristic arc-shaped fluorescein staining pattern. Knowledge of this problem led to the development of larger lenses by Bausch & Lomb and its competitors and is responsible for the generally accepted clinical criterion that soft lenses be fitted such that the lens fully covers the cornea.

Eventually, with the assistance of feedback from eye care practitioners, most soft contact lens manufacturers settled on lens parameters consisting of one or two diameters, ranging from 13.5 mm to 14.5 mm, and one to three base curves (posterior central radii) per diameter, depending on how forgiving (flexible) the lens was, a function of the elastic properties of the polymer and the thickness profile of the lens design.

The value of designing soft contact lenses with a posterior peripheral curve also was recognized empirically by contact lens fitters, and manufacturers adopted this feature as a facilitator of better lens movement. Evidence of some lens movement (the actual amount being relatively unimportant) is another generally accepted clinical criterion for satisfactory performance of soft contact lenses. It informs the clinician that the space between the cornea and lens is not sealed off (i.e., *not tight*, in the language of contact lens fitting). Tight lenses tend to trap biologic debris behind the lens, which can cause anterior segment inflammation, especially in the case of extended-wear lenses (Mertz and Holden 1981).

Lens thickness is another important design parameter that evolved over the first decade or so following the introduction of the first soft contact lens in the United States in 1971. The Bausch & Lomb 12.5-mm lenses had center thicknesses ranging from 0.12 mm to 0.18 mm. Low-water-content HEMA lenses in these thicknesses caused considerable hypoxia-related problems (corneal edema) when worn on a daily-wear basis. It was only after so-called ultrathin lenses (center thickness of 0.06–0.07 mm) were introduced in the middle to late 1970s that hypoxia problems became manageable for a sizable portion of the daily-wear population. In 1977, the Hydrocurve thin lens (Soft Lenses, Inc. San Diego, CA) was the first such lens introduced to the U.S. market, followed shortly by the Bausch & Lomb U3 series lens.

Corneal hypoxia re-emerged as a major problem with the introduction of extended-wear lenses, especially during the overnight phase of extended wear (Holden et al. 1983), when the oxygen available to the cornea is so much less. Efforts to reduce the thickness profiles of soft lenses, even in high-water-content materials, reached the limits of lens manufacture and polymer durability without meeting established critical oxygen requirements (Holden and Mertz 1984).

Disposable-Lens Designs

Beginning in 1987, the designs of disposable contact lenses introduced in the United States did not differ appreciably from the designs of their conventional extended-wear counterparts. Early on, however, the FDA required that manufacturers design their disposable lenses by using parameters that distinguished them from their own conventional soft lenses. Table 5.1 lists the first three disposable lenses introduced in the United States, with their available parameters as of this writing. Although several other disposable lenses have been introduced since then, the products shown in Table 5.1 accounted for nearly 50% of disposable lens new fits in the United States in 1996 (data from Health Products Research [HPR]).

Development of Contact Lens Manufacturing

Molded Sclerals

The earliest glass contact lenses either were ground and polished from glass blocks or were cut from blown glass bubbles (Mandell 1988). In the early 1930s, Dr. Joseph Dallos developed a method of producing glass scleral contact lenses by using a colloidal impression of the anterior ocular surface (after a number of intermediary steps) to produce a brass die for molding the back surface of the lens from molten glass.

Table 5.1 First Disposable Contact Lenses Introduced in the United States

	SeeQuence (Bausch & Lomb, Rochester, NY)	NewVues (CIBA Vision, Duluth, GA)	ACUVUE (Johnson & Johnson, Jacksonville, FL)
Polymer	Polymacon	Vifilcon A	Etafilcon A
Manufacturing process	Spincasting	Cast molding	Stabilized soft molding
Water content	38.6%	55%	58%
Food and Drug Administration polymer group	1 Low water, nonionic	4 High water, ionic	4 High water, ionic
Power range (D)	Plano to −9.00	+4.00 to −10.00	−0.50 to −9.00 (−0.50 to −11.00 in 8.8-mm base curve) +0.50 to +8.00
Diameter/base curve (mm/mm)			
Minus	14.0/8.7*	14.0/8.4 14.0/8.8	14.0/8.4 14.0/8.8 14.4/9.3
Plus		Same as minus	14.4/9.1
Center thickness (mm) @ −3.00 D	0.035	0.06	0.07

*Aspherical spincast back surface equivalent to 8.7-mm spherical base curve.
Source: Data from TTT Tyler. Disposable lenses—clear or visibility tinted sphericals. Tyler's Quarterly Soft Contact Lens Parameter Guide 1995;12:4.

The front surface of the lens then was ground and polished. Preformed glass scleral lenses were also used to fit patients, representing the beginning of the trial method of fitting contact lenses (Sabell 1989).

Even after PMMA became the contact lens material of choice in the late 1930s, scleral lenses with molded back surfaces, either preformed or made from anterior ocular surface impressions, dominated the field. One important change that occurred during the same period was the adoption of lathe cutting as the technique of choice for fabricating the front surfaces of the lenses.

Lathing

Lathing (also known as *turning*) has been used extensively in the manufacture of PMMA corneal lenses, RGP contact lenses, and even hydrogel contact lenses from small cylindrical buttons of polymeric material. In the case of hydrogel lenses, one or both surfaces are turned on a lathe in the dry state before hydration. The advantage of lathing is its versatility. The variety of lens designs that can be produced by this process is nearly limitless; however, the process also has a number of disadvantages. It is labor intensive and, therefore, both expensive and susceptible to significant human error. Also, the lathing process is slow, often taking several days to a week or longer to process a batch of lenses from start to completion. For hydrogel lenses, which are lathed in the dry state, this processing time is a source of error. Atmospheric water vapor (humidity) always is gradually, yet relentlessly, hydrating (swelling) any hydrophilic material when it is in a state of hydration less than its final water content. This creates a moving target for the manufacturer during the dry-state processing of hydrogel lenses. Manufacturers take steps, in varying degrees, to minimize this change, such as environmental humidity control (which cannot be held much below 35% without adversely affecting employee comfort); use of finger cots and masks by employees to minimize the effects of moisture from the skin and breath; and nightly storage of work in process in drying ovens. This phenomenon cannot be eliminated, however, and always has a significant effect on the reproducibility of lathed hydrogel lenses to a degree that depends on the speed of dry-state manufacturing. It also has a major impact on the cost of manufacturing.*

Although the development of automated lathes has reduced some of these problems to a degree, other aspects of the process (polishing, blocking, edging) continue to be sources of error. A totally automated lathing process for hydrogel contact lenses has yet to be developed. Therefore, lathing remains impractical for the mass production of the kind of high-quality, inexpensive contact lenses required for disposable and frequent-replacement products.

Manufacture of Disposable Contact Lenses

A major driving force behind the development of disposable lenses was the fact that, in the 1980s, manufacturing technology leaped ahead of polymer technology. Mass production processes either were developed or were improved to allow for the fabrication of contact lenses in high volume and accurately as well as inexpensively. These three attributes—volume, accuracy, and cost—are the keys to the disposable-lens concept. The manufacturing processes for disposable contact lens products include spincasting (Bausch & Lomb SeeQuence and Occasions); spincast front, lathed back (Bausch & Lomb SeeQuence 2); cast molding (CIBA Vision NewVues and Bausch & Lomb New Day); and stabilized soft molding (Johnson & Johnson ACUVUE and 1•DAY ACUVUE).

Spincasting. After several unsuccessful attempts to produce HEMA contact lenses by casting in closed molds, Professor Otto Wichterle decided to try centrifugal casting in open molds. As a polymer chemist, Wichterle was familiar with centrifugal casting as a technique used to form polymeric thin films (Mandell 1988). He chose to adapt this technique to spinning curved molds. Using glass molds and a mechanical construction kit borrowed from his children, he built the first contact lens spincasting apparatus in his own kitchen (Mandell 1988; Heitz 1989). The molds were spun on an axle driven by a dynamo fashioned from his son's bicycle (later using the motor from a phonograph). The device was completed on Christmas Eve in 1961 and, by New Year's Eve, Wichterle had completed the patent application for the spincasting of HEMA lenses.

---

*To illustrate this point, suppose the *on-target* power yield for a lathing operation is 25% (which would not be unusual). Of course, the overall power yield will be substantially higher because manufacturers of lathed lenses measure the power of every finished lens to find the 25% that came out on target. Instead of discarding the other lenses, however, lenses that are not too far off power (typically, ±1.00 D) will be packaged with labels indicating the power as measured. The labor required to measure the power of every lens is a significant burden to the cost of manufacturing. Although the packaged off-target lenses add to the overall yield, they bloat the company's inventory with unneeded powers. This predicament adds to the cost of inventory, makes controlling inventory unpredictable, and increases the chance for back orders. A well-engineered mass production process, on the other hand, will achieve on-target power yields that approach 100%. Instead of having to measure the power of all lenses, the power of an entire lot can be verified with a small statistical sample. Inventory is much easier to control because it is predictable and can be maintained at minimal levels without fear of back orders.

The rights to the spincasting process followed the same route as the rights to the HEMA material (i.e., purchase by the NPDC and licensure to Bausch & Lomb). Even though Wichterle and his colleagues managed to commercialize spincast HEMA contact lenses in parts of Europe in the early 1960s, the lenses would have fared poorly in comparison with even the earliest lenses produced and marketed by Bausch & Lomb. Credit must be given to a talented team of engineers at Bausch & Lomb who developed the process acquired from Wichterle through the NPDC to a world-class manufacturing process. For at least a decade after the market launch of Bausch & Lomb's Soflens (polymacon) contact lens in 1971, no other manufacturer could compete with the reproducibility and unit cost of lenses produced by the company's spincasting process.

The spincasting process is used to produce Bausch & Lomb's SeeQuence disposable contact lens and Occasions, a polymacon daily-disposable lens being test-marketed as of this writing. The process currently used to produce these modern disposable lenses remains essentially unchanged from the process developed and perfected by Bausch & Lomb in the 1970s.

Spincast Front, Lathed Back.   In the mid-1980s, apparently as a result of declining popularity of its spincast contact lens products, Bausch & Lomb developed its Optima line of premium daily-wear and extended-wear conventional soft contact lenses. This move was accomplished by reengineering a process originally developed in the early 1970s to produce lenses for the international market, which was slow to accept spincast lenses. This revised process, sometimes referred to as *reverse process III* or *RP III*, forms the front surface by spincasting HEMA slowly and polymerizing it in the mold, producing a blank. The posterior surface is then lathed and polished to complete the lens.

Later, Bausch & Lomb employed this process to produce the Medalist lens, the first product introduced exclusively for use on a daily-wear, frequent-replacement basis. The process is also used to manufacture the company's second-generation disposable-lens product, SeeQuence 2.

Cast Molding.   Cast molding is used extensively in many industries to manufacture plastic goods in a cost-effective manner. The process casts liquid plastic monomer between two molds and polymerizes the monomer to form the desired item. Then the two molds are broken apart, and the item is processed for packaging and sale.

The first contact lens company to receive FDA approval for a cast-molding contact lens manufacturing process was American Hydron (Woodbury, NY) in November 1980 (Bailey 1981). American Hydron was owned by the NPDC, the company that brought the Czechoslovakian soft contact lens technology to the United States and sublicensed it to Bausch & Lomb. The NPDC formed American Hydron in 1978, electing to enter the contact lens market in the United States after Bausch & Lomb agreed to relinquish its exclusive license to the technology in favor of a paid-up worldwide nonexclusive license. American Hydron used the cast-molding process to produce low-water-content polymacon lenses, claiming that the new process increased its production capacity ten-fold without requiring additional labor (Anonymous 1981). In 1983, the NPDC sold the company to Allergan, Inc., a major producer of contact lens care products.

When CIBA Vision purchased the contact lens division of American Optical in 1985, it acquired vifilcon A, a 55%-water-content polymer used to produce Softcon, a conventional lathed-lens product. Also acquired in the transaction was a cast-molding manufacturing process that American Optical used to produce a low-water-content daily-wear lens called *AO Superthin.* After transferring the American Optical technology to its facilities in Norcross, GA, CIBA integrated the cast-molding process with the vifilcon A material to launch its disposable contact lens product, NewVues, in 1989, and its daily-wear, frequent-replacement product, Focus, 2 years later.

In 1993, Bausch & Lomb received FDA approval for a new patented cast-molding process called *Form Cast*. In 1994, the company announced that this process would be part of a highly automated and fully integrated manufacturing and inventory control system called *Performa*, developed in collaboration with IBM's Microelectronics Division and scheduled for completion in 1995 (Anonymous 1994a). Indeed, the first product produced with this process, SofLens66, was introduced in mid-1995. SofLens66 is a 66%-water-content lens originally recommended for daily wear and replacement every 2 weeks or less (Anonymous 1995a). (It was approved for disposable extended-wear use in late 1996.) The process also produces New Day, the company's second daily-disposable polymacon lens that, along with the spincast Occasions lens, is being test marketed at this writing (Anonymous 1995b).

Stabilized Soft Molding. In 1981, the giant health care company Johnson & Johnson entered the contact lens field by acquiring Frontier Contact Lenses, a small manufacturer based in Jacksonville, FL. In 1984, the contact lens company, subsequently renamed *Vistakon*, purchased the rights to a patented Danish contact lens manufacturing technology known as *stabilized soft molding* (SSM).

SSM is a form of cast molding, but it has features that differentiate it from the cast-molding processes mentioned earlier. Ordinarily, hydrogel lenses are produced in a dry (prehydrated) state and then hydrated. During hydration, the dry polymer absorbs water, expanding like a sponge, until equilibrium is reached at the polymer's final water content. During hydration, dry manufacturing errors are magnified in proportion to the degree of expansion. The higher the final water content, the greater is the expansion; therefore, errors that fall within dry-manufacturing tolerances may satisfy final hydrated-lens quality standards for low-water-content hydrogels but would be less likely to meet the standards for high-water-content hydrogels. For this reason, the higher the water content of a hydrogel polymer, the more difficult and expensive it is to control the quality and reproducibility of the contact lenses produced.

The primary advantage of the SSM process is that it allows higher-water-content hydrogel lenses to be produced with minimal expansion on hydration. In fact, the expansion is less than that of most low-water-content lenses. This feature is accomplished by adding an inert diluent to the initial monomer formulation. During polymerization, the diluent occupies space that will be replaced later by water. When the lens is hydrated, the diluent is extracted (flushed out), and water takes its place. The net result is that hydration occurs with only minimal expansion.

After acquiring the Danish technology, Johnson & Johnson engineers incorporated many process improvements as SSM development progressed through pilot and scale-up phases. Their efforts advanced state-of-the-art contact lens manufacturing to never-before-achieved levels of production capacity, quality control, and per-unit cost. Since 1987, SSM has been used to manufacture ACUVUE, the first FDA-approved disposable contact lens. The process also is used to manufacture Johnson & Johnson's daily-wear 2-week replacement lens, SUREVUE. More than any other single factor, SSM has been responsible for the company's success in building the disposable-lens business. In 1994, more contact lenses were produced by SSM than by all the other contact lens manufacturing processes combined throughout the world.

Although key elements in the SSM process are controlled by computer-aided automation systems, a large portion of the process remains heavily dependent on human labor. On a per-lens basis, labor is the largest single contributor to the cost of manufacturing. For instance, before final packaging, optical comparators that magnify lenses more than 10 times are used by specially trained and carefully audited technicians to inspect every finished lens for flaws or cosmetic imperfections. Another major cost contributor is mold procurement. The molds are supplied by a vendor who manufactures them in another part of the United States and therefore they must be shipped to the company's Florida manufacturing plant; also, large inventories have to be warehoused, and extensive quality assurance procedures have to be performed. Not only is the repetitive handling costly in terms of labor, but it also generates a certain amount of damage to the molds, resulting in a lower yield.

In 1990, Johnson & Johnson made the decision to develop a daily-disposable contact lens. To undertake such a challenging project, the company had to commit enormous amounts of capital and human resources to develop a second-generation manufacturing process that would be capable of lowering manufacturing costs enough to make the wearing of up to 730 lenses per year affordable to patients. By early 1993, the company's engineers had succeeded, once again, in advancing state-of-the-art contact lens manufacturing. The result of their efforts was a totally automated, continuous-flow process called *MAXIMIZE*, in which the entire SSM process is fully integrated in the form of stand-alone production modules. Depending on demand, modules can be placed in or out of service to increase or decrease production capacity as needed to meet demand and to control inventory. Major cost reductions were achieved by producing molds and primary packaging (blister packs) on-line, by optimizing polymerization and hydration times, by using conveyors and part-handling robotics to move lenses continuously through the process, by inspecting finished lenses with a computerized high-resolution video image analysis system, and by hundreds of other improvements. The MAXIMIZE process now produces Johnson & Johnson's daily-disposable product, 1•DAY ACUVUE, continuously from mold production to final secondary packaging in 30-lens multipacks untouched by human hand. The process lowers per-lens manufacturing cost to a level at which labor is replaced by depreciation as the largest single cost contributor.

DEVELOPMENT OF DISPOSABLE CONTACT LENSES

Evolution of the Disposable-Lens Concept

The idea of a disposable soft contact lens is nearly as old as the soft lens itself, going all the way back to the inventor, Otto Wichterle. According to Sabell (1980), as Wichterle and his colleagues were developing a production-model spincasting machine in the early 1960s, they conceived of the idea of disposable lenses, believing that the reproducibility and low cost of spincasting would make it economically feasible for patients to replace their lenses after short intervals. It is not clear whether they considered disposability because of the fragility of the lenses they were producing in those days, as suggested by Sabell (1980); because they recognized the potential problems posed by surface spoilation; or both.* They were never able to

---

*In an interview conducted in the early 1980s (Bailey et al. 1987), Wichterle was asked what advice he had for dealing with soft contact lens deposits. His answer: "Discard the coated lenses and replace them with new ones. What we need is an inexpensive, absolutely reproducible lens so the [replacement lens] will not require another fitting."

proceed beyond the concept stage, however, because mounting development costs severely limited their options, and there was no incentive once the technology was licensed to the Americans.

As experience with hydrogel contact lenses increased throughout the late 1970s and early 1980s, it became clear that the problem of long-term surface spoilation presented a serious impediment to successful wear for many patients. Clinical sequelae, ranging from mild to severe and from chronic to acute, included reduced vision, ocular irritation, allergic reactions, inflammation and, occasionally, infection.

Hydrogel lens spoilation is not preventable, no matter how heroic the measures taken by patients or practitioners. The hydrophilicity of a hydrogel lens gives it an affinity for nearly anything attracted to or soluble in water, leading to the inevitable surface buildup of the substances listed earlier (see footnote on page 70) to clinically unacceptable levels. At best, this process is slowed by careful surfactant and enzymatic cleaning. It is well documented, however, that most patients comply very poorly with proper lens care and maintenance procedures (Collins and Carney 1986; Chun and Weissman 1987; Lakkis and Brennan 1994).

The aforementioned clinical sequelae occur with both daily-wear and extended-wear hydrogels, although to a greater degree with extended-wear lenses. Compared with full-time daily-wear lenses, extended-wear lenses worn full time remain in contact with ocular tissue two to three times longer and are cleaned and disinfected only approximately one-seventh as often. Even though the contact lens industry has invested enormous amounts of capital and labor in the attempt to develop spoilation-resistant polymers, the results to date have been disappointing. In the late 1970s and early 1980s, with no breakthrough materials on the development horizon, interest in alternative approaches gathered momentum.

Although the disposable-lens idea was conceptually simple and attractive, the job of making it a reality certainly was not. Manufacturing costs and other problems made implementation technically and economically unfeasible for more than two decades after Wichterle and his colleagues first pondered the idea.* Various approaches have been devised for limiting the rapidity of spoilation, including powerful in-office cleaners, all sorts of abrasives from homemade sodium bicarbonate slurries to contact lens polishing compounds (e.g., X-pal), and a surfactant cleaner with polymeric beads, but over the long term, such efforts usually have proved to be more effective at destroying lens surfaces than at preventing surface spoilation.

In 1987, one trade journal editor wrote, "Since 1978, *collagen* and *disposable* have been synonymous terms in the contact lens field" (Bailey et al. 1987). He was referring to an interview conducted in 1978 with Dr. O. A. Battista of Fort Worth, TX, who was developing a collagen lens called the *Landel lens* (Anonymous 1979). Dr. Battista described his invention as a "throw-away lens," claiming it had the feature of self-obsolescence. After a certain period (2 months being mentioned in the interview), the lens was supposed to turn cloudy, indicating to the patient that it was time for a replacement. Updates on the progress (or lack thereof) of the collagen lens were reported from time to time during the next 8 years (Bailey 1979, 1981, 1984; Bailey et al. 1987). Battista eventually licensed the technology to the French company Essilor. Another collagen lens reportedly was under development by American Hydron from 1979 to

---

*Actually, from the late 1970s on, the opportunity probably was available for Bausch & Lomb to pioneer the disposable lens concept by leveraging the low cost and reproducibility of lenses produced by its spin-casting technology but, other than its FreshLens spare lens program, described later in this section, the company took no steps in this direction.

1987 (Bailey 1984; Bailey et al. 1987). Expectations were elevated in anticipation of a collagen lens because of the potential its high water content (90% or greater) had for increasing oxygen transmission to the cornea. Unfortunately, as far as this author has been able to determine, no collagen lens ever has reached the marketplace. The exact reason for this situation never has been documented adequately, although rumor has it that the material was unstable, possibly owing to a tendency to dissolve in the presence of certain human tear enzymes (perhaps the very mechanism of its self-obsolescence).

In the late 1970s and early 1980s, unlike the experience in most of Europe, extended-wear soft contact lenses remained relatively popular in Scandinavia. At that time, the most popular extended-wear lens in Sweden was the Scanlens, a 71%-water-content hydrogel lens. The development of the Scanlens was a collaborative effort between Klas Nilsson, a Gothenberg optician and contact lens manufacturer, and two very prolific British polymer scientists, Dr. Donald Highgate and John Frankland. Highgate and Frankland invented several other well-known contact lens materials of the time, including Sauflon and Duragel. In an interview (Anonymous 1983), Nilsson noted that extended-wear patients made up approximately 50% of his contact lens practice and that it had been his experience that "red eyes and giant papillary conjunctivitis [were] seldom seen" due to the fact that his extended-wear patients replaced their lenses regularly at 6-month intervals "before trouble starts." He developed marketing and distribution programs that provided his patients with financial and other incentives to comply with his instructions. He was influential with his fellow Swedish practitioners, most of whom were Scanlens customers, and encouraged them to adopt these programs for their patients. The approach caught on and became widely accepted not only in Sweden but in other parts of Scandinavia where Nilsson's lenses were not even available.

Another version of the disposable-lens concept was Bausch & Lomb's FreshLens program (Schwartz 1986), introduced in late 1985. Practitioners were given the option of enrolling their extended-wear patients in this program if the patients wore Bausch & Lomb O3 or O4 series lenses. Two weeks after the lenses were dispensed, Bausch & Lomb would mail to enrolled patients a second pair of lenses in glass vials marked "left" and "right," along with instructions and tweezers for removing the lenses from the vials. Three months after the original dispensing, patients were sent a reminder to replace their initial lenses with the spare pair and to return the worn pair to Bausch & Lomb in the now empty vials. At 6 months, patients were sent a notice to return to their practitioner for a follow-up visit. At the follow-up visit, patients received two new lenses, if deemed appropriate by their practitioner, and the cycle was repeated. Patient noncompliance (failure to return the lenses) was reported to the practitioner. Later, the program was expanded to include other Bausch & Lomb products, including daily-wear lenses. Acceptance of the FreshLens program was mixed because many practitioners were reluctant to release the home addresses of their patients to a company.

In the early 1980s, the personal computer revolutionized manufacturing technology in many industries, including the contact lens industry. Major advances in state-of-the-art contact lens manufacturing occurred and, before long, Bausch & Lomb's spincasting was no longer the only mass production process in the industry capable of producing large quantities of highly reproducible soft contact lenses at low per-unit cost.

Development of the First Disposable Lens

The disposable lens introduced by Johnson & Johnson originated in Scandinavia. Klas Nilsson's notion that "better" extended wear was achievable with high-water-content lenses replaced every 6 months probably influenced Danish ophthalmologist and entrepreneur Dr. Michael Bay, who was responsible for developing the Danalens. This lens is believed to be the first commercial product marketed as a disposable contact lens, more or less as we know the concept today—that is, as multiple individually packaged lenses (multipacks) (Bailey et al. 1987; Barnhart and Chun 1993). Bay needed a manufacturing process to produce his disposable lenses and collaborated with a group of Danish engineers. The fruit of their labor was the invention of the original SSM process.

Although the commercial success of the Danalens was modest at best, attempts to sell the technology did generate interest, particularly among the large American manufacturers. The technology was primitive, however, and had serious shortcomings, including an undercured polymer, primary packaging that tended to leak, poor optics, and extremely poor edges. In the end, all the major contact lens manufacturers backed away, but the management at Johnson & Johnson became intrigued by the disposable lens, possibly recognizing its conceptual commonality with so many of the company's other products. Whatever the reason, Johnson & Johnson purchased the technology in 1984. Johnson & Johnson's decision to proceed with the development of the disposable lens was a defining moment, destined to have a profound and lasting effect on how contact lenses are prescribed and worn in the 1990s.

Johnson & Johnson encountered many obstacles during the disposable-lens development effort. Some have been mentioned (see Stabilized Soft Molding). A separate but related obstacle was the discovery that the original Danalens polymer was unstable over time and had to be replaced. The company was fortunate that its one and only substitution option worked. That material, etafilcon A, a 58%-water-content material, had just received extended-wear approval from the FDA in a product called *Vistamarc,* no longer produced.

Another obstacle, the question of contamination, arose when it was learned that the Danalens packaging was not always airtight (Benjamin et al. 1985), probably as a result of damage induced during high-pressure autoclave sterilization. Traditionally, soft contact lenses have been packaged in glass vials, sealed with silicone rubber stoppers held in place with crimped aluminum caps. A different packaging approach was needed for disposable lenses because glass vials were cumbersome, heavy, expensive, and reusable, an undesirable feature for a disposable lens.* The Danalens was packaged in "eight-packs" (plastic strips with eight compartments, each containing a lens in packing solution, sealed with foil covers). Johnson & Johnson retained the idea of nonreusable plastic, or "blister," packs, but a new airtight design had to be developed and tested thoroughly to overcome the problem. The company also adopted a different overall approach by packaging each lens in a small individual blister pack that was easy to carry in a pocket or purse. Lenses were shipped in secondary packages called "multipacks," each containing six blister packs, a 6- or 12-week supply for one eye, depending on whether prescribed for 1- or 2-week replacement.

Not all the obstacles encountered were of a technical nature. For instance, in the absence of any precedent, the disposable lens raised formidable regulatory questions that had to be resolved with the FDA. Another (and perhaps the biggest) obstacle was overcoming contact lens practitioners' concerns over the disposable concept: their natural aversion to dispensing multiple pairs of lenses without verifying clinical

---

*This problem preceded the idea of daily-wear frequent-replacement lenses.

performance beforehand and their skepticism about the likelihood of their patients discarding their lenses as instructed.

Eventually, all obstacles were overcome, and Johnson & Johnson introduced the ACUVUE Disposalens contact lens shortly after receiving FDA approval in December 1986 (the term *Disposalens* later was dropped). The product initially was test-marketed in Florida, where little excitement was generated. Changes and adjustments were made on the basis of what was learned. One key change was a lower price; another was the idea of complimentary diagnostic lenses to encourage practitioners to try disposable lenses on patients who might benefit from them. The test marketing was resumed, this time in California as well as in Florida, with very positive results. The ACUVUE lens finally was released nationwide in the United States in June 1988, marking the beginning of a new era in contact lens prescribing.

It was not long before the ACUVUE lens was joined by competitors. By the end of the same year, Bausch & Lomb was test marketing its first disposable product, called *SeeQuence*, a spincast polymacon lens. By the spring of 1989, CIBA Vision started test-marketing a disposable product called *NewVues*, a cast-molded, 55%-water-content (vifilcon A) lens. Other companies were caught off guard by the rapidly growing popularity of disposable lenses, and by the time they initiated their own disposable-lens development programs, the early market entries were dominating the most rapidly (and perhaps only) growing segment of the contact lens market.

Defining a Disposable Lens

This seemingly trivial pursuit is not accomplished as easily as it might seem. There has been, and continues to be, confusion about what a disposable lens is and what it is not. Some clarification is useful.

The FDA defines a disposable lens as one worn only once (single use) and then thrown away, never to be used a second time. This definition seems simple enough. Today, only two modalities of wear satisfy the FDA definition: (1) *weekly-disposable*, defined as single-use extended wear of up to 7 days/6 nights, with the lens discarded immediately on removal, and (2) *daily-disposable*, defined as single use of up to 1 day during waking hours only, with the lens discarded immediately on removal at the end of the day before sleep. Single use is the feature held in common by these two modalities, qualifying them both as true disposable lenses. When worn on a single-use basis, disposable lenses do not require cleaning and disinfecting.

In the real world, however, other forms of contact lens wear are called *disposable*. In some countries, for instance, the term *disposable* is used commonly to describe contact lens replacement of 1 month or less, regardless of whether the lenses are worn on a single-use basis or are reused any number of times ranging from twice to every day of the month. In the United States, the most commonly used definition of disposable lens connotes any contact lens replaced within 2 weeks or less, regardless of wearing habit. The reason for this choice is that market research companies (most notably HPR) now report industry sales figures using this as their definition of *disposable.*

Confusion arises when manufacturers promote the disposable-lens convenience advantage of not requiring any cleaning or disinfecting. Of course, the company is referring only to single use of disposable lenses, for which the claim is true. However, patients wearing contact lenses on a daily-wear reusable basis with 2-week or monthly replacement may think that they are wearing disposable lenses. Obviously, such patients place themselves at risk if somehow they reach the conclusion that, as wearers of "disposable lenses," they can stop cleaning and disinfecting their lenses.

Another confusing issue is the role of cleaning. It may seem illogical to patients, or even to practitioners, to have to clean lenses that will be discarded in such a short time. Thinking disinfecting alone is enough, they may opt to eliminate cleaning from the regimen. Often they are unaware that cleaning is an important element in the disinfection "system." Without the cleaning process, most modern disinfecting solutions are relatively ineffective and leave the lens vulnerable to major microbial challenge.

The existence of these confusing issues only underscores the importance of the practitioner-patient relationship in ensuring that patients are instructed and informed properly about such matters.

Frequent Replacement

Practitioner attitudes toward extended wear have varied widely, although most who have engaged in extended-wear fitting in recent years have prescribed disposable lenses. Of those willing to prescribe extended-wear lenses regularly, some do so indiscriminately, whereas others carefully screen and closely follow their patients, knowing that extended wear is not suitable for everyone. Others prescribe extended-wear lenses only reluctantly at the insistence of their patients; still others refuse to fit extended-wear lenses at all.

It was not long after disposable lenses were introduced that some practitioners began to realize, either because they did not want to prescribe extended-wear lenses for any of their patients or because a patient was not a good candidate for extended wear, that disposable lenses could be worn on a daily-wear basis and still offer the benefit of preventing spoilation problems. They started prescribing ACUVUE lenses for daily wear, with regular replacement usually every 2 weeks. The emergence of this second disposable-lens modality was unanticipated. It was obvious that contact lenses worn this way were not true disposable lenses according to the FDA definition, and eventually the term *frequent replacement* evolved to categorize planned-replacement lenses worn on a reusable daily-wear basis, which now includes products that have been developed and marketed intentionally for this purpose, with recommended replacement intervals ranging from 2 weeks to 6 months. As mentioned earlier, a daily-wear lens that is replaced every 2 weeks or less is now often referred to as *disposable* for market-trend analysis purposes.

Because the ACUVUE lens was being prescribed so often for daily wear, Johnson & Johnson took the necessary steps to obtain FDA approval for a daily-wear indication, which was received in 1990. In 1989, however, Bausch & Lomb introduced the polymacon Medalist lens, which was recommended for monthly replacement and was the first contact lens developed specifically to be marketed as a daily-wear frequent-replacement product. Later, CIBA Vision developed a monthly frequent-replacement lens called *Focus*, and Johnson & Johnson introduced a thicker, easier-to-handle lens called *SUREVUE* for daily-wear 2-week replacement.

The obvious advantage of the frequent-replacement category of planned-replacement lenses is the lower risk of physiologic problems with daily wear than with extended wear. Of course, the trade-off for this is that frequent-replacement lenses must be cleaned and disinfected before every re-use. Some advantage can be claimed over conventional daily-wear lenses, however, because multipurpose care systems generally can be used. Multipurpose systems are simpler to use and, as such, are thought to promote better patient compliance. A more tangible advantage for frequent replacement of up to 1 month is that enzymatic cleaning usually is not required.

Misconceptions

When used properly, disposable and frequent-replacement lenses offer a number of important advantages (Table 5.2). From the point of view of ocular health, these advantages are linked to prevention of long-term contact lens spoilation, and it does not seem unreasonable to think of fitting disposable and frequent-replacement lenses as a form of preventive medicine. Studies support the contention that disposable and frequent-replacement lenses offer a better way to wear both extended-wear and daily-wear soft contact lenses, respectively, with fewer complications, fewer symptoms, and fewer unscheduled problem visits to the practitioner when compared with conventional lenses (Boswall et al. 1993; Poggio and Abelson 1993a, b; Nilsson and Montan 1994a, b).

The development of disposable lenses was driven by growing concerns in the mid-1980s over reports of corneal ulcers associated with extended-wear contact lenses. The Contact Lens Institute study reported that extended-wear lenses were associated with a risk of ulcerative keratitis 5–15 times higher than that associated with daily-wear lenses (Schein et al. 1989), although the absolute risk (incidence) was shown to be quite low for both modalities* (Poggio et al. 1989).

As mentioned, when disposable lenses were introduced in 1987, they were recommended for single-use extended wear of up to 1 week. Used in this fashion, there is no need for a cleaning and disinfecting regimen, a common source of microbial contamination. It was predicted that by eliminating the need for a care regimen, disposable lenses would reduce the higher risk of ulcerative keratitis reported in the Contact Lens Institute study for conventional extended-wear soft lenses. Unfortunately, as logical as this seemed at the time, it was a misconception. It has been shown since that the risk of ulcerative keratitis for disposable extended-wear lenses is comparable to that for conventional extended-wear lenses (Schein et al. 1994), although conventional extended-wear lenses may be associated more often with sight-threatening infectious microbial ulcers, and disposable extended-wear lenses with sterile peripheral corneal ulcers of immunologic origin (Donshik 1993; Poggio and Abelson 1993a; Slack 1993; Nilsson and Montan 1994a, b).

The widely held misconception—that disposable lenses do not have to be cleaned—(discussed in Defining a Disposable Lens) is a serious problem and deserves further mention. The idea that no cleaning is necessary is true only for single-use disposable lenses. Any reuse of a soft contact lens, even if it is called a disposable lens, requires that the lens be cleaned every time it is removed if it is going to be used again, because cleaning is the key element in disinfecting the lens.

Another often-voiced misconception about disposable lenses is that they have superior oxygen transmission properties compared with conventional soft contact lenses and that hypoxia problems do not occur with disposable lenses. As previously discussed (see footnote on page 72), the oxygen transmissibility of a hydrogel contact lens depends on its water content and thickness. It is true that most disposable lenses have been designed to optimize oxygen transmissibility as much as possible. Several of the disposable lenses currently available do meet (or come close to meeting) the established critical oxygen requirements for daily-wear lenses (Fatt 1997), but none meet the critical oxygen requirements for extended-wear lenses (Holden and Mertz 1984). In terms of corneal

---

*The often-quoted ulcerative keratitis annualized incidence figures of 4.1 per 10,000 for daily-wear lenses and 20.9 per 10,000 for extended-wear lenses also mean that in any given year, 99.96% of daily-wear patients and 99.79% of extended-wear patients do not develop ulcerative keratitis.

Table 5.2 Benefits of Disposable and Frequent-Replacement Contact Lenses

---

Any clinical benefit derived from prevention of long-term lens spoilation
    Consistent high-quality vision and comfort that do not degrade over time
    Fewer contact lens complications
    Fewer contact lens symptoms
    Fewer unscheduled visits; less chair time
Any clinical benefit derived from simpler contact lens care and maintenance
    If worn on single-use basis only
        Ultimate convenience of no care and maintenance requirement
    If worn on reusable basis
      Can usually use multipurpose (all-in-one) solutions for cleaning* and disinfecting
        Advantages
            More convenient (one solution does all)
            Better compliance (simpler instructions)
            Fewer toxicity and sensitivity reactions (milder preservatives)
      Enzymatic cleaning usually not required
Better patient control
    If patient picks up contact lenses in the office: opportunity to check progress, address problems,
      and reinforce compliance issues
    If patient finds office pick-up inconvenient: direct shipment from manufacturer possible
      (varies by country and manufacturer)
Greater patient satisfaction; more referrals
Fewer patient dropouts
Spare lenses always available to patient if needed
Complimentary diagnostic lenses
    Easy and cost-effective fitting
    Possibility for a free trial offer (lenses) to potential patients
    Possible use to assist patients in selecting spectacle frames
    Possible use as substitutes for patient's regular lenses on order or backorder
    No need for in-office diagnostic lens disinfection
Reversible alternative to refractive surgery

---

*Cleaning never can be eliminated for reused lenses, even if lenses are reused for 2 wks or less, because cleaning is an essential element in disinfecting any contact lens. Proper carrying-case hygiene also is essential.

hypoxia response, no difference should be expected between a disposable extended-wear lens and a conventional extended-wear lens if their oxygen transmissibility is equal.

Daily-Disposable Contact Lenses

Since their introduction, the use of disposable and frequent-replacement contact lenses has experienced spectacular growth, mostly at the expense of conventional extended-wear and daily-wear lenses. The experience has been more of a redistribution of existing patients to planned replacement than an expansion of the overall contact lens population. During most of the 1980s and the early 1990s, the contact lens industry experienced virtually no growth, because the number of new contact lens patients each year was offset by an equal number of dropouts. The population of contact lens wearers did begin to grow again in 1993. Disposable and frequent-replacement lenses probably were responsible for most of the growth, more likely as a result of reducing the number of dropouts rather than of expansion of the number of new wearers. Both modalities involve compromises that leave room for improvement and that limit their potential for attracting nonwearers. Single-use disposable lenses offer the convenience and compliance advantages of not having to be cleaned and disinfected, but these advantages are offset by the inherent problems associated with extended wear. Frequent-replacement lenses eliminate the problems of extended wear but must be cleaned and disinfected every time they are reused. As a result of these compromises, many potential patients continue to reject contact lenses as either too risky or too much trouble.

At the beginning of this decade, in considering how to overcome the factors limiting growth of the contact lens population, the question in the minds of many in the industry was "How can contact lenses be improved enough to attract spectacle wearers and former contact lens dropouts?" The obvious answer was to develop extended-wear lenses capable of being worn continuously and remaining complication-free for at least a month. Surveys say that this type of product is what potential contact lens patients really want.

In 1990, the goal of a safe, 30-day extended-wear contact lens was elusive, and it continues to be so at this writing. At Johnson & Johnson, however, a second option emerged. Dr. Hikaru Hamano, who has the largest contact lens practice in the world, advised Johnson & Johnson that extensive clinical experience and research had convinced him of the need for disposable lenses that could be replaced every day. Other experts agreed and, as a result, the company committed to development of a daily-disposable contact lens product.

With daily-disposable wear, new lenses are placed on the eyes every day, worn only during waking hours, and then are removed and discarded before sleep, never to be worn a second time. They combine the best features of disposable and frequent-replacement lenses—true single-use disposability and daily-wear safety, respectively—and avoid the undesirable features that have limited the two modalities from reaching their potential (the problems of extended wear and the inconvenience of cleaning-disinfecting, respectively).

Beginning in 1990, a new contact lens–manufacturing process was developed that, when completed 3 years later, advanced state-of-the-art contact lens manufacturing to levels of production capacity, precision, and per-unit cost never achieved before. The process, called *MAXIMIZE*, is described in greater detail in the section Stabilized Soft Molding.

In parallel with the development of the MAXIMIZE process, a prospective clinical investigation was initiated in an attempt to show to practitioners and their patients clinical evidence of the benefits of daily lens replacement.

This 3-year study (Solomon et al. 1996) compared the clinical performances of 229 subjects randomly assigned to daily-disposable wear, frequent-replacement wear, or conventional daily wear. The results support the hypothesis that daily-disposable wear offers clinical advantages compared with the other wearing modalities. Compared with conventional daily wearers, daily-disposable wearers were more likely to be asymptomatic; reported fewer symptoms of redness, cloudy vision, and grittiness/dirty sensation; reported better subjective vision and overall satisfaction; and had fewer lens surface deposits, complications, tarsal abnormalities, and unscheduled visits. Compared with 1- to 3-month frequent-replacement wearers, daily-disposable wearers reported fewer symptoms of foreign body sensation, redness, cloudy vision, and grittiness/dirty sensation; reported better subjective vision, comfort, and overall satisfaction; and had fewer surface deposits, complications, and tarsal abnormalities. Compared with 2-week frequent-replacement wearers, daily-disposable wearers reported better subjective vision and better overall satisfaction and had fewer surface deposits and tarsal abnormalities.

These results are consistent with a study conducted in Japan and involving 23,000 patients (Hamano et al. 1994) that compared the complication rate of daily-disposable lenses with the rates of various other types of contact lenses (including PMMA lenses, RGP lenses, acryl elastomers, high- and low-water-content daily-wear hydrogels, and weekly extended-wear disposable lenses). With a high degree of statistical certainty, daily-disposable lenses were shown to have the lowest complication rate of all the types studied.

Other studies conducted with daily-disposable lenses (Kame et al. 1993; Farkas 1994; Kame 1994; Nilsson and Soderquist 1995) all lead to the same general conclusion: Daily-disposable wear appears to be the healthiest, most convenient, and most trouble-free form of contact lens wear yet developed.

The daily-disposable modality became a reality in 1993 when a test market was initiated with the first such product, 1•DAY ACUVUE. Later that year, Bausch & Lomb began test-marketing its own daily-disposable product, a spincast polymacon lens called *Occasions.*

In August 1994, Johnson & Johnson launched its product in the western region of the United States. A Scottish company, Award plc, had also developed a daily-disposable lens (73%-water-content, cast-molded) called *Premiere* (Anonymous 1994b), which was launched in the United Kingdom in late 1994. One aspect of the technology used to produce this lens was novel in that the lens was molded in what eventually became part of the lens package. This feature undoubtedly lowered the cost of production but raised some concern about the adequacy of extracting potentially toxic unpolymerized monomer from the final lens (Sariri et al. 1995).

In 1995, Bausch & Lomb began test-marketing its second daily-disposable lens, New Day, in four states: Iowa, Illinois, Wisconsin, and Minnesota (Anonymous 1995c). This product, another polymacon lens, is produced by the company's new automated cast-molding process developed in collaboration with computer giant IBM (described in more detail in the section, Cast Molding). It is not clear at this writing whether the New Day lens is meant to replace or to supplement the Occasions lens also being test-marketed. In early 1996, Bausch & Lomb acquired its third daily-disposable product when it purchased the Scottish company Award plc.

In February, 1995, Johnson & Johnson launched the 1•DAY ACUVUE lens nationwide in the United States, Canada, Japan, and the United Kingdom. Based on performance to date, the future of daily-disposable lenses appears to be very bright. Demand for the product has exceeded all expectations, delaying launching of the product in other countries and postponing expansion of the number of available lens parameters. The lens already has captured 2.7% of the daily-wear spherical lens new fits and 4.1% of all disposable-lens new fits in the United States (data from HPR fourth quarter 1996 results). In late 1996, CIBA Vision began test marketing a daily-disposable product called *Dailies* in Norway. A list of all daily-disposable contact lenses known as of this writing is provided in Table 5.3.

A New Paradigm: Shorter Is Better

In recent years, the disposable and frequent-replacement segments of the contact lens market have experienced spectacular growth and a proliferation of new products. With the introduction of the ACUVUE disposable lens in 1987, Johnson & Johnson pioneered an entire new category of soft contact lenses that have had a revolutionary effect on the contact lens market, in the sense that other companies have been forced to develop their own disposable and frequent-replacement lenses to remain compet-

Table 5.3 Daily-Disposable Contact Lens Products

	Premiere (Award plc; Bausch & Lomb, Rochester, NY)	Occasions (Bausch & Lomb)	New Day (Bausch & Lomb)	Dailies (CIBA Vision, Duluth, GA)	1·DAY ACUVUE (Johnson & Johnson, Jacksonville, FL)
Country of origin	Scotland	United States	United States	United States	United States
Polymer	No USAN name	Polymacon	Polymacon	Nelfilcon A	Etafilcon A
Manufacturing process	Cast molding	Spincasting	Cast molding	Cast molding	Stabilized soft molding
Water content	73%	38.6%	38.6%	69%	58%
Food and Drug Administration polymer group	2 High water, nonionic	1 Low water, nonionic	1 Low water, nonionic	2 High water, nonionic	4 High water, ionic
Power range (D)	−0.25 to −6.50	−0.50 to −6.00	−0.50 to −6.00	−0.50 to −6.00	−0.50 to −9.00 +0.50 to +6.00
Diameter/base curve (mm/mm)	14.4/8.7	14.0/8.7*	14.0/8.7	13.8/8.6	14.2/9.0 14.2/8.5
Center thickness (mm) @ −3.00 D	0.14	0.043	0.043	0.10	0.07

USAN = U.S. Adopted Names.
*Aspherical spincast back surface equivalent to 8.7-mm spherical base curve.
Source: Most of the data are from TTT Tyler. Disposable sphericals. Tyler's Quarterly Soft Contact Lens Parameter Guide 1994;12:4; TTT Tyler. Disposable lenses—clear or visibility tinted sphericals. Tyler's Quarterly Soft Contact Lens Parameter Guide 1995;12:4; and M Guillon, L McGrogan, JP Guillon, et al. Effect of material ionicity on the performance of daily disposable contact lenses. Contact Lens and Anterior Eye 1997;20:in press.

itive. The ACUVUE lens has become the most prescribed contact lens, not only in the United States but also in the world, and as of this writing, it is marketed in 67 countries. Some attribute this success to marketing hype, but that reasoning would not explain sustained growth of these categories for 8 years with no signs of slowing. The explanation for this success lies in the improvement in clinical response resulting from preventing soft contact lenses from developing spoilation problems. Patients have recognized the difference, and they have told their practitioners who have told the industry that there is value in this approach to contact lens wear.

In 1995, for the first time, the total number of disposable and frequent-replacement new fits in the United States exceeded the number of conventional lens new fits. There appears to be no going back: A shift in the soft contact lens paradigm has occurred, from what might be characterized as the old "make-it-last" model of the 1970s and 1980s to the new "shorter-is-better" model of the 1990s. With the growing popularity of daily-disposable lenses, the paradigm may be about to shift once again, this time to a shortest-is-best model. It remains to be seen whether history can repeat itself.

REFERENCES

Anonymous. Coming attraction: the throw-away lens. Contact Lens Forum 1979;4(2):21.

Anonymous. Hydron cast molding approved. Contact Lens Forum 1981;6(1):9.

Anonymous. Closing the gaps in soft lens history. Contact Lens Forum 1982;7(6):27.

Anonymous. Preventing extended wear problems, the Swedish way. Contact Lens Forum 1983;8(3):21.

Anonymous. Bausch & Lomb announces agreement with IBM to bring the next generation of soft contact lenses to market. Bausch & Lomb Press Release, June 15, 1994a.

Anonymous. Daily disposables set for UK launch. Optician 1994b;208(Aug 18):6.

Anonymous. Bausch & Lomb SofLens66 high-water non-ionic disposable contact lens. MDDI RE-PORTS—The Gray Sheet August 14, 1995a;25.

Anonymous. A 'New Day' dawns in contact lens convenience. PR NEWSWIRE Today's Headlines, Story 32261, March 13, 1995b.

Anonymous. The daily disposable alternative. Contact Lens Spectrum 1995c;10(3):5.

Bailey NJ. Contact lens update. Contact Lens Forum 1979;4(3):25.

Bailey NJ. Update report 1981. Contact Lens Forum 1981;6(2):19.

Bailey NJ. Contact lens update, 1984. Contact Lens Forum 1984;9(2):31.

Bailey NJ, Sposato P, Barr JT. The contact lens—past, present and future. Contact Lens Spectrum 1987;2(7):17.

Barnhart LA, Chun MW. Disposable Hydrogel Contact Lens Systems (Chapter 57). In ES Bennett, BA Weissman (eds), Clinical Contact Lens Practice. Philadelphia: Lippincott, 1993;1.

Barr JT, Bailey NJ. History and Development of Contact Lenses (Chapter 11). In ES Bennett, BA Weissman (eds), Clinical Contact Lens Practice. Philadelphia: Lippincott, 1993;1.

Benjamin WJ, Bergmanson JPG, Estrada PJ. Disposable "eight-packs." Int Eyecare 1985;1:494.

Boswall GJ, Ehlers WH, Luistro A, et al. A comparison of conventional and disposable extended wear contact lenses. CLAO J 1993;19:158.

Chun MW, Weissman BA. Compliance in contact lens care. Am J Optom Physiol Opt 1987;64:274.

Collins MJ, Carney LG. Compliance with care and maintenance procedures amongst contact lens wearers. Clin Exp Optom 1986;69:174.

de Carle J. Hydrophilic Lenses for Continuous or Extended Wear. In M Ruben (ed), Soft Contact Lenses: Clinical and Applied Technology. New York: Wiley, 1978;199.

Donshik PC. Corneal ulcers and disposable extended wear lenses. CLAO J 1993;19:8.

Dreifus M. The Development of pHEMA for Contact Lens Wear. In M Ruben (ed), Soft Contact Lenses: Clinical and Applied Technology. New York: Wiley, 1978;7.

Efron N, Pearson RM. Centenary celebration of Fick's *Eine Contactbrille*. Arch Ophthalmol 1988;106:1370.

Farkas B. Raising contact lens safety to a new level. Optom Today, 1994;2(6):31.

Fatt I. The FDA challenge to developers of extended wear contact lenses. Optician 1977;173(Mar 18):10.

Fatt I. Oxygen Transmission. In OH Dabezies (ed), Contact Lenses—The CLAO Guide to Basic Science and Clinical Practice (2nd ed). Boston: Little, Brown, 1989;10.1.

Fatt I. Comparative study of some physiologically important properties of six brands of disposable hydrogel contact lenses. CLAO J 1997;23:49.

Feinbloom W. A plastic contact lens. Am J Optom Arch Am Acad Optom 1937;14:14.

Fick AE. A contact spectacle [English translation by CH May]. Arch Ophthalmol 1888;17:215.

Grant T, Terry R, Holden BA. Extended wear of hydrogel lenses—clinical problems and their management. Probl Optom 1990;2:599.

Hamano H, Watanabe K, Hamano T, et al. A study of the complications induced by conventional and disposable contact lenses. CLAO J 1994;20:103.

Hart DE. Deposits and Coatings: Hydrogel Lens/Tear-Film Interactions (Chapter 33). In ES Bennett, BA Weissman (eds), Clinical Contact Lens Practice. Philadelphia: Lippincott, 1993;1.

Heitz RF. History of Contact Lenses. In OH Dabezies (ed), Contact Lenses—The CLAO Guide to Basic Science and Clinical Practice (2nd ed). Boston: Little, Brown, 1989;1.1.

Herschel JFW. Light: XII. Of the Structure of the Eye and of Vision. In Encyclopedia Metropolitana, Vol. 4. London: 1845;398.

Hodd NFB. An analysis of permanent wear success. Optician 1977;174(July 1):23.

Hofstetter HW. Leonardo's contact concept. Contact Lens Forum 1984;9(12):15.

Hofstetter HW, Graham R. Leonardo and contact lenses. Am J Optom Arch Am Acad Optom 1953;30:41.

Holden BA, Mertz GW. Critical oxygen levels to avoid corneal edema for daily and extended wear contact lenses. Invest Ophthalmol Vis Sci 1984;25:1161.

Holden BA, Mertz GW, McNally JJ. Corneal swelling response to contact lenses worn under extended wear conditions. Invest Ophthalmol Vis Sci 1983;24:218.

Kame RT. Are your patients ready for daily disposable? Contact Lens Spectrum 1994;9(9):26.

Kame RT, Farkas B, Lane I, et al. Patient response to disposable contact lenses worn on a daily disposable regimen. Contact Lens Spectrum 1993;8(6):45.

Kelly C. Backfire on FDA extended-wear guidelines. Contact Lens Forum 1977;2(9):57.

Knoll HA. William Feinbloom: pioneer in plastic contact lenses. Contact Lens Forum 1977;2(8):29.

Knoll HA. The first plastic lens. Contact Lens Forum 1979;4(7):80.

Lakkis C, Brennan NA. Non-compliance with contact lens care and maintenance procedures. Optom Vis Sci 1994;71(Suppl):13.

McEachern CL, Cannon WM, McClay MC. Cosmetic extended wear: a positive view. Contact Lens Forum 1982;7:19.

McKechnie JL (ed). Webster's New Universal Unabridged Dictionary (2nd ed). New York: Simon & Schuster, 1983;449, 863.

Mandell RB. Historical Developments. In RB Mandell (ed), Contact Lens Practice (4th ed). Springfield, IL: Thomas, 1988;5.

Mertz GW, Holden BA. Clinical implications of extended wear research. Can J Optom 1981;43:203.

Müller A. Brillenglaser und Hornhautlinsen [spectacle lenses and contact lenses]. Inaugural dissertation, Kiel, Germany: University of Kiel, 1889.

Nilsson SEG, Montan PG. The hospitalized cases of contact lens–induced keratitis in Sweden and their relationship to lens type and wear schedule: results of a three-year retrospective study. CLAO J 1994a;20:97.

Nilsson SEG, Montan PG. The annualized incidence of contact lens–induced keratitis in Sweden and its relationship to lens type and wear schedule: results of a 3-month prospective study. CLAO J 1994b;20:225.

Nilsson SEG, Soderquist M. Clinical performance of a daily disposable contact lens: a 3-month prospective study. J Br Contact Lens Assoc 1995;18:81.

Poggio EC, Abelson M. Complications and symptoms in disposable extended wear lenses compared with conventional soft daily wear and soft extended wear lenses. CLAO J 1993a;19:31.

Poggio EC, Abelson M. Complications and symptoms with disposable daily wear contact lenses and conventional soft daily wear contact lenses. CLAO J 1993b;19:95.

Poggio EC, Glynn RJ, Schein OD, et al. The incidence of ulcerative keratitis among users of daily-wear and extended-wear soft contact lenses. N Engl J Med 1989;321:779.

Poster M (moderator). The jury is in: extended wear—a roundtable discussion. Rev Optom 1982;119:37.

Refojo MF. The Chemistry of Soft Hydrogel Lens Materials. In M Ruben (ed), Soft Contact Lenses: Clinical and Applied Technology. New York: Wiley, 1978;19.

Refojo MF. Chemical Composition and Properties. In M Ruben, M Guillon (eds), Contact Lens Practice. London: Chapman & Hall Medical, 1994;23.

Remba MJ. What consumers think about extended wear. Contact Lens Forum 1982;7(11):31.

Sabell AG. The History of Contact Lenses. In J Stone, AJ Phillips (eds), Contact Lenses—A Textbook for Practitioner and Student (2nd ed). London: Butterworth, 1980;1.

Sabell AG. The History of Contact Lenses. In AJ Phillips J, Stone (eds), Contact Lenses—A Textbook for Practitioner and Student (3rd ed). London: Butterworth, 1989;1.

Sariri R, Mann A, Franklin V, Tighe B. Acidic and basic impurities in soft contact lenses. Poster presented at British Contact Lens Association Conference, London, May 1995.

Schein OD, Buehler PO, Stamler JF, et al. The impact of overnight wear on the risk of contact lens–associated ulcerative keratitis. Arch Ophthalmol 1994;112:186.

Schein OD, Glynn RJ, Poggio EC, et al. The relative risk of ulcerative keratitis among users of daily-wear and extended-wear soft contact lenses. N Engl J Med 1989;321:773.

Schwartz CA. Contact lens update 1986 (part 1). Contact Lens Forum 1986;11(1):23.

Slack JW. The increasing proportion of contact lens–associated corneal ulcers [ARVO abstract]. Invest Ophthalmol Vis Sci 1993;34(suppl):1407.

Solomon OD, Freeman MI, Boshnick EL, et al. A 3-year prospective study of the clinical performance of daily disposable contact lenses compared with frequent replacement and conventional daily wear contact lenses. CLAO J 1996;22:4.

Sulaiman S, Holden BA. World contact lens usage. Paper presented at Eighth International Contact Lens Congress, Port Douglas, Australia, September 1993.

Terry RL, Schnider CM, Holden BA, et al. CCLRU standards for success of daily and extended wear contact lenses. Optom Vis Sci 1993;70:234.

Tighe BJ. Contact Lens Materials. In AJ Phillips, J Stone (eds), Contact Lenses—A Textbook for Practitioner and Student (3rd ed). London: Butterworth, 1989;72.

Tripathi RC, Tripathi BJ. Lens Spoilage. In OH Dabezies (ed), Contact Lenses—The CLAO Guide to Basic Science and Clinical Practice (2nd ed). Boston: Little, Brown, 1989;45.1.

Tripathi RC, Ruben M, Tripathi BJ. Soft Lens Spoilation. In M Ruben (ed), Soft Contact Lenses: Clinical and Applied Technology. New York: Wiley, 1978;299.

Wichterle O. The Beginning of the Soft Lens. In M Ruben (ed), Soft Contact Lenses: Clinical and Applied Technology. New York: Wiley, 1978;3.

Zantos SG. Extended Wear Lenses: An Historical Overview (Chapter 54). In ES Bennett, BA Weissman (eds), Clinical Contact Lens Practice. Philadelphia: Lippincott, 1993;1.

Appendix 5.1

Milestones of Modern Contact Lens Development

PREINVENTION MILESTONES

1508   The idea of a contact lens (CL) occurs to Leonardo Da Vinci (unproved).

1823   English astronomer Sir John Herschel authors the first written description of a CL.

INVENTION OF THE CONTACT LENS

1888–1889   The CL is invented independently by:
Swiss ophthalmologist Adolph Eugen Fick
French ophthalmologist Eugene Kalt
German medical student August Müller

MILESTONES PRECEDING DISPOSABLE CONTACT LENSES

	Contact lens materials	Contact lens designs	Contact lens manufacturing
Glass lenses (1888–1939)			
1888	The first CLs are made of glass, the only clear solid substance known at the time. High specific gravity makes them uncomfortable and unstable on the eye. Oxygen impermeability severely limits wearing time.	Corneal design is tried initially (in dispute) but the lens will not stabilize on eye and the design is abandoned quickly. Scleral design distributes weight more evenly, giving greater stability, but seals off cornea from its oxygen supply.	Early glass lenses are ground and polished from glass blocks or cut from blown-glass bubbles.

	Contact lens materials	Contact lens designs	Contact lens manufacturing
1932 (approx.)		Joseph Dallos introduces trial lens fitting with preformed diagnostic CLs.	Dallos casts molten glass to form back surface of scleral CLs, using molds made from eye impressions.

Rigid plastic lenses (1934 to present)

	Contact lens materials	Contact lens designs	Contact lens manufacturing
1934	Polymethyl methacrylate (PMMA) is invented.		
1936	William Feinbloom introduces first plastic-containing CLs (resin scleral flange with central glass optic).		
1938	First PMMA lenses are fitted by Hungarian ophthalmologist Itsvan Gyorrfy.		
1939	PMMA is much lighter than glass, so PMMA lenses are more comfortable and stable on eye than glass but are just as impermeable to oxygen.	Theodore Obrig and Philip Salvatori introduce PMMA CLs in New York City. Early designs mimic glass sclerals. Sealing off cornea from oxygen supply still is a major problem, limiting wearing time. Determined efforts to facilitate oxygen transport behind CLs meet little success. Nevertheless, Obrig and Salvatori's business is a commercial success.	Back surface of PMMA scleral CL is cast in a mold. Mold is either a clone of back surface mold used to make the diagnostic lens selected by trial fitting or is made from impression mold of patient's anterior eye. Front surface is lathed.
1948		Kevin Touhy files patent on first PMMA corneal design, generally regarded as beginning of modern era of CLs. Makes CL wear possible for significant numbers of patients.	PMMA corneal lenses are manufactured from PMMA "buttons" by lathing both surfaces. Buttons are molded individually or cut from molded rods of PMMA.

	Contact lens materials	Contact lens designs	Contact lens manufacturing
1950		George Butterfield files patent for improved PMMA corneal lens design featuring posterior peripheral curve(s) flatter than central radius. Facilitates more movement for greater tear exchange and more oxygen behind lens.	
1970	Norman Gaylord invents the siloxane-methacrylate rigid gas-permeable (RGP) polymer.		
1974	Gaylord patent is issued.		
1978	First RGP material, cellulose acetate butyrate (CAB), is approved by the US Food and Drug Administration (FDA).	First RGP CL product, Danker Lab's Meso CAB lens, reaches U.S. market but fares poorly, owing to polymer instability.	
1979	FDA approves siloxane-methacrylate RGP material.	FDA grants premarket approval to Polycon (siloxane-methacrylate) lens, the first commercially successful RGP product.	

Conventional soft plastic lenses (1954 to present)

	Contact lens materials	Contact lens designs	Contact lens manufacturing
1954	Czechs Otto Wichterle and Drahoslav Lim invent hydroxyethyl methacrylate (HEMA), the original soft CL polymer.		
1961			Wichterle completes spincasting process for manufacturing soft CLs.
1965	National Patent Development Corporation (NPDC) acquires rights to HEMA from Czech government	First soft CL designs are patterned after PMMA corneal lenses but are too small and flexible	Bausch & Lomb acquires rights to spincasting process along with HEMA material from the

	Contact lens materials	Contact lens designs	Contact lens manufacturing
	and sublicenses to Bausch & Lomb.	to stay on cornea. Problem is solved with semiscleral design that extends just beyond the limbus.	NPDC.
1968	The FDA classifies HEMA as a drug, increasing regulatory requirements for approval.		
1970	English optometrist John de Carle develops first high-water-content hydrogel material in quest for continuous-wear CLs.		
1971	Bausch & Lomb receives FDA approval for polymacon (HEMA) material.	Bausch & Lomb receives FDA premarket approval and introduces the Soflens (polymacon) CL, first soft CL in the United States.	FDA approves spin-casting for manufacturing the Bausch & Lomb Soflens CL.
1975		de Carle introduces Permalens, the first "continuous-wear" CL, in the United Kingdom.	
1976	Medical Devices Act of 1976 becomes law. The soft CL is classified as a medical device and no longer as a drug.		
1977		First "ultrathin" soft CL (Hydrocurve) is introduced in the United States. Solves hypoxia-related problems for many marginal patients. Other companies soon follow suit with their own thin soft CLs.	

	Contact lens materials	Contact lens designs	Contact lens manufacturing
1980			American Hydron receives FDA approval for first CL cast-molding manufacturing process.
1981		The FDA approves Permalens and Hydrocurve, first CLs approved for cosmetic extended-wear (30-day) correction of myopia.	
1989		Contact Lens Institute–sponsored study is published and shows that risk of ulcerative keratitis is higher for extended-wear soft CLs than for daily-wear lenses. FDA asks industry to shorten recommended extended-wear period from 30 days to 7 days and 6 nights.	

MILESTONES IN THE DEVELOPMENT OF DISPOSABLE CONTACT LENSES (1963 TO PRESENT)

1963	Wichterle and colleagues, experiencing polymer fragility and spoilation problems with early HEMA CLs, speculate that the low cost and high reproducibility of spincasting could make a disposable lens approach economically feasible. The technology is sold, however, before they can test the theory.
1980 (approx.)	Unlike in most of Europe, extended-wear lenses remain popular in Scandinavia. Some attribute this to the popularity of the high-water-content Scanlens with planned replacement every 6 months.
1984	Johnson & Johnson acquires stabilized soft molding (SSM) technology from Danish entrepreneur and initiates improvement program.
1985	Bausch & Lomb initiates FreshLens program. Extended-wear patients are sent spare pairs of CLs in vials for replacement at 3-month intervals.
1986	Johnson & Johnson receives first FDA approval of a disposable lens, recommended for single-use extended wear of up to 7 days and 6 nights. Called *ACUVUE*, the lens is made of a 58%-water-content material (etafilcon A) already approved for extended wear in 1984 and is manufactured by the SSM process.

1987   Johnson & Johnson introduces the ACUVUE disposable lens by test marketing it first in the state of Florida and later in California.

1988   Johnson & Johnson launches ACUVUE disposable lens nationwide in the United States.

Bausch & Lomb begins test marketing the SeeQuence CL, the second disposable lens introduced in the United States. The lens is made of low-water-content polymacon material and is manufactured by using Bausch & Lomb's 1970s spincasting technology.

1989   A third disposable lens is introduced in the United States. CIBA Vision test markets the NewVues disposable lens, a cast-molded 55%-water-content (vifilcon A) lens.

Bausch & Lomb introduces the Medalist lens, a polymacon lens produced by Bausch & Lomb's RPIII process (spincast front, lathed back) and the first CL marketed specifically as a daily-wear frequent-replacement (monthly) lens.

1990   The ACUVUE lens is approved for daily wear and is recommended for daily-wear 2-week replacement for patients not suited to extended wear.

1993   Johnson & Johnson completes its MAXIMIZE advanced state-of-the-art manufacturing technology, a totally automated version of the SSM process. The process is developed to manufacture Johnson & Johnson's daily-disposable product, 1•DAY ACUVUE, which begins test marketing in two U.S. cities.

1994   Bausch & Lomb begins test-marketing a spincast polymacon daily-disposable CL called *Occasions*.

Johnson & Johnson launches 1•DAY ACUVUE in the western United States.

A Scottish company, Award plc, launches a daily-disposable lens in the United Kingdom. The lens, called *Premiere*, is made of a 73%-water-content material, cast-molded in the lens's final package.

1995   Bausch & Lomb begins test-marketing its second polymacon daily-disposable lens, called *New Day*. The lens is manufactured by a new automated cast-molding process developed by Bausch & Lomb in collaboration with IBM.

Johnson & Johnson launches 1•DAY ACUVUE nationwide in the United States, Canada, Japan, and the United Kingdom.

1996   Bausch & Lomb purchases Award plc, thus acquiring the Premiere daily-disposable lens.

CIBA Vision initiates test marketing of its daily-disposable product, Dailies, in Norway.

6

Extended-Wear Contact Lenses

Claire M. Vajdic and Brien A. Holden

Extended wear is defined as the wearing of contact lenses for 24 hours or longer, including a period of sleep. For the purposes of this chapter, *disposable extended-wear lenses* are defined as lenses that are discarded after 1 or 2 weeks of wear without removal for sleep or cleaning, and *conventional extended-wear lenses* are defined as lenses that are reused on repeated occasions after overnight removal, usually once a week, for cleaning and disinfection.

Disposable extended-wear lenses were introduced as a way of avoiding the adverse ocular effects associated with lens deposits and lens aging. The concept of regular lens replacement has been accepted widely, and disposable lenses now represent approximately 45% of new soft lens fittings in the United States (Barr 1997).

Clinical experience and in vitro investigations with conventional hydrogel lens extended wear have reinforced the theoretical advantages of disposable extended-wear lenses. Conceptually, regularly replaced lenses should reduce the complications associated with lens deposits and lens aging and remove potential problems associated with care systems. Disposable extended-wear lenses, however, are essentially the same as conventional extended-wear lenses in terms of material composition, oxygen transmissibility, and lens design. Therefore, the advantages of disposable lenses, as compared with conventional lenses, are derived from frequent lens replacement rather than from any inherent superiority in the lens material itself.

Extended wear of contact lenses has long been the goal of patients, practitioners, and manufacturers. In one survey, 97% of prospective patients expressed the desire to be able to wear their lenses continuously for at least 6 nights per week (Holden 1989). The ultimate contact lens, at least for most wearers, is one that can be worn safely and comfortably, provides excellent vision, and does not have to be removed at all.

Nevertheless, extended wear of hydrogel lenses has been fraught with difficulties. Complications such as hypoxia, inflammation, and serious infections have dogged the products that were introduced in the mid-1970s and 1980s. Because the disposable-lens wear schedule limits exposure of the eye to soiled and contaminated lenses, it was hoped that these lenses would provide safe, long-term, extended wear, despite the reservations of physiologists concerning chronic problems related to hypoxia.

Practitioners and researchers have found, however, that safe extended wear is not yet a reality with currently available soft lenses, even when they are used on a disposable basis. An understanding of the inflammatory processes that occur during overnight wear and the pathogenesis of contact lens–associated corneal infection has yet to be achieved. In addition, many of the mechanisms underlying morphologic and functional changes induced by extended hydrogel lens wear are understood poorly. Essential ocular requirements, such as true surface compatibility, also are not met with currently available hydrogel extended-wear systems. Lacking this fundamental knowledge, and in the absence of a truly biocompatible system, frequent replacement of lenses is the most favorable option available to maximize ocular health over the long term.

Extended wear is prescribed for the correction of ametropia (cosmetic extended wear) and also for aphakia and therapeutic purposes. This chapter concentrates on issues associated with cosmetic wear, although the basic principles elaborated here are applicable to all forms of lens use. The structural and functional changes and inflammatory reactions induced by hydrogel lens extended wear are discussed and compared for disposable and conventional lenses. Hypoxia and corneal infection are covered only briefly, as Chapters 2 and 10 are dedicated to these issues.

HYPOXIA

Corneal Oxygen Requirements and Metabolism

In the open eye, the atmosphere is the primary source of oxygen for the cornea. Other sources include the aqueous humor, particularly for the endothelium and posterior stroma, and the tarsal and limbal vasculature. When the eye is closed, oxygen is supplied mainly via the vasculature of the tarsal conjunctiva, which provides twice as much oxygen as does the aqueous humor under these conditions. Essential corneal metabolites are provided by the limbal vasculature, aqueous humor, and tear film.

The oxygen demands of the cornea are very high and are increased further during eye closure, owing to the rise in temperature and subsequent increase in the metabolic rate of the epithelial cell layer (Freeman and Fatt 1973). Farris et al. (1965) reported that the oxygen uptake rate of the epithelium is higher than that of the stroma or the endothelium. This finding was confirmed partially by Freeman (1972), who determined the relative oxygen consumption rates of the epithelium to stroma to endothelium to be 2 to 2 to 1, respectively.

Contact lens wear interferes with the transfer of atmospheric oxygen to the cornea, thereby creating hypoxia, increasing anaerobic metabolism, and reducing glycogen stores within the epithelium. Glycolysis and reduced consumption of protons lead to increased lactate production. These changes are thought to induce the imbibement of fluid through the epithelium into the interfibrillar spaces in the stroma, leading to stromal swelling (i.e., corneal edema; Davson 1972). There is a linear relationship between corneal hydration and corneal thickness. Contact lens wear also decreases the oxygen tension and increases the lactate concentration within the aqueous humor that bathes the endothelium (Hamano et al. 1975; Mikami et al. 1981; Kamiya et al. 1982).

Hamano et al. (1983) suggested that the minimum precorneal level of oxygen required to maintain aerobic epithelial metabolism is 13%. Other investigators have shown that precorneal oxygen tension can be reduced to approximately 10% before there is a measurable increase in corneal thickness (Holden et al. 1984). The best estimate of the minimum epithelial oxygen requirement is likely to be 15%, however, as reported by both Mizutani et al. (1983) and Williams (1986).

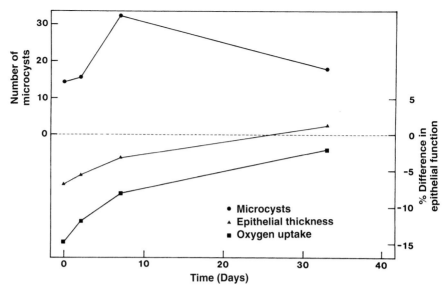

Figure 6.1 Changes in epithelial oxygen uptake, epithelial thickness, and numbers of epithelial microcysts after cessation of long-term wear of high-water-content hydrogel contact lenses. The dotted line represents the control eye data. (Reprinted with permission from BA Holden, DF Sweeney, A Vannas, et al. Effects of long-term extended contact lens wear on the human cornea. Invest Ophthalmol Vis Sci 1985;26:1489.)

Even short-term lens wear affects corneal oxygen consumption. This finding may be linked to the suppression of basal epithelial cell mitosis during lens wear (Hamano et al. 1983). Hill (1965) observed that the epithelial oxygen uptake rate increases following short-term lens wear, yet recovers within 60 seconds of lens removal. Farris et al. (1971) demonstrated significant increases in oxygen uptake after 6–8 weeks of hydrogel lens daily wear. In contrast, Carney and Brennan (1988) showed a reduction in oxygen uptake below baseline levels after approximately 19 weeks of daily hydrogel lens wear.

Holden et al. (1985a) reported a 15% reduction in epithelial oxygen uptake rate after long-term hydrogel extended lens wear. Oxygen consumption rate required up to 33 days' cessation of lens wear to return to normal levels (Figure 6.1). The authors hypothesized that decreased oxygen consumption is the result of either a decrease in aerobic metabolic activity or a reduction in the number of epithelial cells.

It also has been shown that hydrogel lens wear decreases the transepithelial potential, although not to the same extent as does hard lens wear (Hamano et al. 1976; Kwok 1983). These investigators suggested that edema may inhibit epithelial ion transport. Huff (1990) demonstrated, however, that edema does not result from inhibition of epithelial or endothelial ion transport mechanisms.

Holden et al. (1981) proposed that overnight corneal swelling during hydrogel lens wear results from a combination of factors, including hypoxia, an unidentified "lens effect," and increased corneal temperature. Other possible contributing factors may include carbon dioxide accumulation, tear film pH and hypotonicity, mechanically induced alterations in corneal metabolism, and inflammation (Sweeney 1991).

Even with the eyes open, contact lens wear impedes the efflux of carbon dioxide from the cornea and post-lens tear film (Holden et al. 1987). Bonanno and Polse (1987a) provided evidence that lens wear induces stromal acidosis at a greater rate and to a greater extent than can be attributed to hypoxia alone. This effect is due to the contribution of carbonic acid, which forms within the stroma as a result of the accumulation of carbon dioxide. This finding is relevant also to epithelial cellular function because several studies have demonstrated the role of pH in the control of glycolysis, membrane ion secretion, and mitotic activity.

In summary, it is clear that contact lens wear induces significant metabolic compromise within the cornea. The direct effects of hypoxia and stromal acidosis are unchanged by regular lens replacement. Indeed, the effects of hydrogel lens spoilation on oxygen transmissibility are negligible (Huth et al. 1984). Where hypoxia is a component of a multifactorial etiology, lens-related complications often are reduced but are not eliminated totally by lens replacement. Regular (particularly overnight) lens removal may minimize the suppression of corneal aerobic metabolism, however.

No studies have compared directly the metabolic effects resulting from conventional-lens versus disposable-lens extended-wear schedules. Nevertheless, statistical analysis of study variables by Holden et al. (1985a) identified three factors that contribute to reduced epithelial oxygen uptake rate during hydrogel lens wear: thicker lenses, less mobile lenses, and fewer lens removals each month.

Overnight and Residual Corneal Edema

Mandell and Fatt (1965) were the first to report an increase in corneal thickness during sleep without lens wear, later measured to be approximately 4%. This normal physiologic response is short lived, however, and corneal thickness returns to baseline levels within 1 hour of eye opening. Corneal swelling during continuous wear of current hydrogel lens materials also is cyclic, reaching approximately 12% overnight and 4% during the day (Holden et al. 1983). This indicates that the cornea deswells by a maximum of 8% after eye opening with lenses in place (Figure 6.2). Therefore, the authors recommended that during extended wear, overnight edema be held to a maximum of 8% to allow the cornea to reattain normal thickness during the day. They also noted that individuals with thicker corneas exhibited significantly more edema during extended wear, perhaps due to a lower level of oxygen diffusion from the aqueous humor.

Many investigators have observed significant individual variations in the levels of open- and closed-eye response to hypoxia. Suggested contributing factors include individual differences in corneal and crystalline lens oxygen requirements, endothelial structure and function, tear chemistry, lid action, lens pumping, and physiologic lagophthalmos. Aphakic eyes exhibit a significantly lower corneal swelling response compared with phakic eyes, possibly owing to reduced epithelial oxygen uptake rate and a thinner epithelium or increased efflux of lactic acid from the cornea (Holden et al. 1982). Additionally, clinical impression has suggested that older individuals are better suited to extended wear than are younger individuals, although statistical analysis has not supported this observation (Koetting et al. 1988; Sweeney 1991). An age-related reduction in corneal metabolic rate could play a role in such a trend.

Zantos (1981) reported that the overnight swelling response decreases with greater duration of continuous hydrogel lens wear. Since then, several studies also have suggested adaptation in the stromal edema response during extended wear. Polse et al. (1990) measured in vivo hydration control and proposed that the effect of lens wear on corneal hydration control was dose dependent.

Recently, Solomon (1996) reported that patients who exhibit corneal swelling of 5% or less within 2 hours of awakening from overnight hydrogel lens wear are sig-

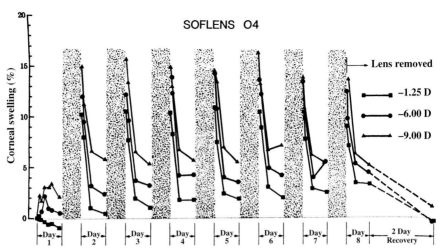

Figure 6.2 Corneal swelling versus time for 10 unadapted subjects wearing Bausch & Lomb (Rochester, NY) Soflens O4 series contact lenses continuously for a period of 1 week. (Reprinted with permission from BA Holden, GW Mertz, JJ McNally. Corneal swelling response to contact lenses worn under extended wear conditions. Invest Ophthalmol Vis Sci 1983;24:218.)

nificantly less likely to experience signs and symptoms indicative of significant residual corneal edema over a period of 7 nights of extended wear.

Nonsteroidal anti-inflammatory drugs have been suggested as a treatment for lens-induced edema. There is no evidence to support their usefulness in conjunction with currently available conventional or disposable hydrogel lenses in the short or long term, however (Efron 1986).

During extended wear, detection of corneal effects related to hypoxia requires careful and precise examination of the cornea on a number of occasions, including within 1 hour of eye opening. The difficulties inherent in this approach, together with individual variations in edema response, may underlie the discrepancies observed among various studies in the incidence of hypoxic complications for different lens types. Residual corneal edema was not reported by Nilsson and Lindh (1990) in their evaluation of extended and flexible wear of disposable lenses over a 6-month period. Similar negative findings also were noted by Gruber (1988) and Woods (1989). Donshik et al. (1988) reported signs of corneal edema in four of 733 patients evaluated. In contrast, Ivins (1988) reported seven discontinuations due to edema in a 39-patient disposable-lens extended-wear study. On the basis of measured lens oxygen transmissibility, these latter findings are likely to be more accurate.

Kotow et al. (1987a) reported that corneal swelling was not affected by regular lens replacement. Further clinical studies at our institution (Cornea and Contact Lens Research Unit, Sydney, Australia) have shown that conventional and disposable extended-wear hydrogel lenses of similar oxygen transmissibility induce a similar level of overnight and residual corneal edema (La Hood et al. 1988).

Contact Lens Transmissibility

The blink-mediated tear pump makes an insignificant contribution to corneal oxygenation during extended wear of hydrogel lenses. Contact lens oxygen transmissibility is the primary factor affecting the supply of oxygen to the corneal surface. Lens oxygen transmissibility (Dk/L) is dependent on the diffusivity (D) and solubility (k) of oxygen in the material, and lens thickness (L). For current hydrogel contact lens materials, the diffusivity and solubility of oxygen in the material are dependent largely on the water content of the material (Refojo and Leong 1979). For other contact lens materials, such as silicone elastomer and rigid-lens polymers, oxygen transmissibility is a function of the structural characteristics of the material and is not related to water content.

Holden and Mertz (1984) determined that a lens Dk/L of 87×10^{-9} Dk units (1 Dk unit = $10^{-10} \times cm^3$ [STP] $\times cm^2/cm^3 \times$ sec mm Hg = 1 barrer) was required to limit lens-induced overnight corneal edema to the "no-lens" level of 4%. A hydrogel material has yet to be developed that meets this criterion and thereby avoids generating anaerobic corneal metabolism during overnight lens wear. A Dk/L of 34×10^{-9} Dk units was proposed by Holden and Mertz as a compromise minimum requirement. Such a lens would induce 8% overnight edema and allow recovery to zero edema during the day. Unfortunately, no current hydrogel lens is able to satisfy even this compromise criterion.

Excess carbon dioxide (hypercapnia) can also be a problem, and therefore, carbon dioxide transmissibility is also an important prerequisite for extended wear. There is an association between oxygen transmissibility and carbon dioxide transmissibility, and the relative transmissibility of materials to carbon dioxide is greater than that of oxygen (Ang and Efron 1989).

In terms of avoiding corneal hypoxia and hypercapnia, the future lies in the refinement of novel lens polymers with transmissibilities that are not limited by the water content (hydration) of the material. With these new hydrogel materials, oxygen and carbon dioxide gas would permeate through the polymer in addition to the aqueous phase of the material (Refojo 1996). Consequently, these materials would have a higher oxygen transmissibility than standard hydrogel materials of similar hydration. Currently, the oxygen transmissibilities of various conventional and disposable extended-wear lens types are similar: approximately 10×10^{-9} to 20×10^{-9} Dk units (Weissman et al. 1991).

STRUCTURAL EFFECTS OF EXTENDED WEAR

Acute and chronic, transient and irreversible changes in the morphology of all corneal layers have been documented with extended wear of hydrogel lenses. Generally, it is believed that the majority of these changes are related to chronic corneal hypoxia, although stromal acidosis also may be a significant factor. These morphologic changes often result in functional changes. Alterations in the structure of the limiting layers of the cornea—the epithelium and the endothelium—pose the greatest risk during hydrogel lens extended wear.

Corneal Epithelium

Corneal Staining and Other Corneal Surface Phenomena

In addition to compromising the corneal epithelium via hypoxia, lens wear also provides the opportunity for mechanical and biochemical disruption of the anterior epithelial layers, evidenced clinically as corneal staining. There are a number of known causes of staining during lens wear: edema, hypoxia, lens deposits, lens care products, lens fit, lens surface or edge irregularities, foreign bodies, improper lens insertion or removal, tear film disruption, and accumulated metabolic waste products.

Such lens-related complications as toxic keratitis and superior limbic keratopathy typically are attributable to preservatives in lens care products. The reuse of conventional extended-wear lenses promotes the adsorption and release of these compounds by the lens polymer itself or by deposits on the lens surface. Regular lens replacement should avoid or significantly reduce these complications.

The physical presence of a contact lens on the eye disrupts the spreading of the tear film over the corneal surface and the exchange of tears beneath the lens. Because a significant proportion of hydrogel lenses adhere to the corneal surface during overnight wear (Kenyon et al. 1988), the increased pressure, accumulation of debris, and disruption of the mucous layer would be expected to increase the risk of epithelial compromise.

A nonmechanical cause of corneal staining may involve chemical alteration of the structures that support the epithelium, including the tear film. O'Leary et al. (1985) noted that the rate of epithelial desquamation is controlled by the level of calcium in the precorneal tear film. In vitro studies conducted by Bachman and Wilson (1985) demonstrated that specific levels of potassium and other ions (e.g., calcium, magnesium, phosphate, bicarbonate, and sodium) in the precorneal tear film are required to maintain the integrity of corneal epithelial cells.

Future studies of tear biochemistry may provide more information about the relationship between the tear film and the corneal surface, in particular the structure and composition of the glycocalyx, and the impact of hydrogel lens wear. An understanding of this complex structure is important for determining the cause of the breakdown of the corneal epithelial barrier. An intact epithelium is necessary to prevent corneal invasion by most pathogenic organisms, such as *Pseudomonas aeruginosa*, the bacterium most commonly isolated from patients exhibiting contact lens–related infectious keratitis.

The incidence of corneal staining during hydrogel lens extended wear is unclear. Nilsson and Lindh (1990) and Donshik et al. (1988) reported a low incidence of corneal staining during extended and flexible overnight wear of disposable lenses. Efron and Veys (1992) suggested that the prevalence of edge defects is greater in disposable lenses than it is in conventional lenses. These investigators reported that edge defects on ACUVUE (Johnson & Johnson, Jacksonville, FL) disposable lenses induced a statistically significant increase in corneal staining after 6 hours of lens wear, although the clinical significance of this finding was unclear. A retrospective comparison of disposable-lens extended wear and conventional-lens extended wear by Boswall et al. (1993) identified a lower occurrence of superficial punctate corneal staining with disposable-lens wear. The average wearing time for the disposable-lens wearers was significantly shorter than that of the conventional-lens wearers, however, which may have contributed to the result. It is evident that there is some controversy regarding the incidence of corneal staining during extended wear of disposable and conventional hydrogel lenses.

Rapid and marked epithelial disruption and corneal staining have been reported with various hyperthin, high-water-content hydrogel lenses designed to provide more oxygen to the cornea than hydrogel lenses of standard parameters (Efron et al. 1986; Holden et al. 1986a; Zantos et al. 1986; Orsborn and Zantos 1988) (Figure 6.3). These studies demonstrated that for current hydrogel lens polymers, lens thickness

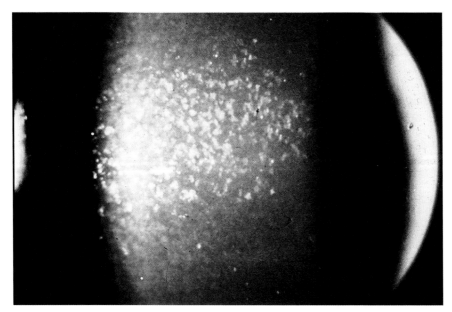

Figure 6.3 Slit-lamp photograph of epithelial disruption and corneal staining induced by lens dehydration during wear.

cannot be reduced beyond a critical level because of significant lens dehydration and subsequent disruption of the epithelial cells. Therefore, highly permeable nonhydrogel lenses are required to meet the oxygen demands of the cornea without compromising the corneal epithelium. Current highly permeable nonhydrogel materials such as silicone elastomer induce clinically unacceptable corneal staining associated with lens adherence and surface hydrophobicity, however, and their use is limited to the correction of aphakia in infants and children.

In 1974, Millodot demonstrated decreased corneal sensitivity with hydrogel lens wear (Millodot 1974); this effect was found later to be the result of hypoxia (Millodot and O'Leary 1980). In addition, O'Leary and Millodot (1981) found that lens wear, particularly hydrogel lens wear, significantly reduces the damage threshold of the peripheral cornea. Also, they found that the threshold for damage to the superficial epithelium without lens wear is lower than the sensation threshold (Millodot and O'Leary 1981). These findings suggest that the threshold interval between sensation and damage may be increased further during lens wear. As a result, corneal damage during lens wear may go unnoticed by the patient, thereby increasing the risk of further complications. There have been no studies comparing the corneal sensitivity or damage threshold of those who wear conventional and disposable hydrogel lenses. Because changes in corneal sensation are a consequence of corneal hypoxia, however, it is unlikely that there would be any differences.

Epithelial adhesion is considered to be essential for maintenance of the epithelial barrier function. Studies in animal models by Madigan et al. (1987) and Madigan and Holden (1992) demonstrated that extended wear of conventional hydrogel lenses reduces the adhesion of the corneal epithelium to the underlying layers, owing to a reduction in the number of hemidesmosomes, one of the epithelium-basement membrane attachment systems (Figure 6.4). Suggested mechanisms for this phenomenon include mechanical deformation of basal cell shape and hypoxia-induced increases in

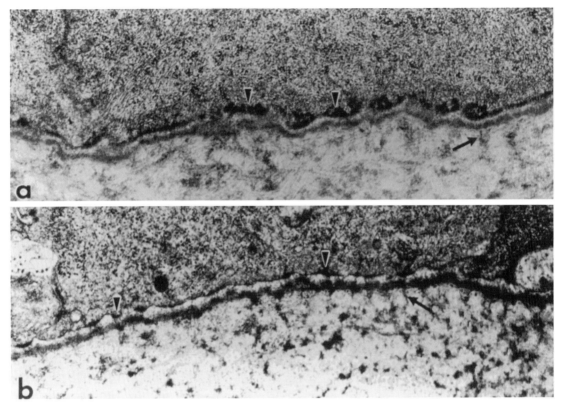

Figure 6.4 Electron micrographs from control (a) and lens-wearing cat corneas showing the epithelial basement membrane region (b). In the control cornea (a), hemidesmosomes are obvious along the basement membrane and occur in chains (arrowheads). After 30 days of contact lens wear (b), the hemidesmosomes are reduced in density and appear as single, discrete units (arrowheads). Anchoring filaments are visible adjacent to hemidesmosomes in both corneas (arrows). (Original magnification ×28,300.) (Photograph by Michele Madigan, Cornea & Contact Lens Research Unit, University of New South Wales, Sydney, Australia.)

intracellular calcium; hence, this morphologic change would be expected to be induced by disposable-lens extended wear as well.

Lemp and Gold (1986) used wide-field color specular microscopy to monitor epithelial morphology during extended wear of conventional hydrogel lenses and identified further changes of significance in epithelial barrier function. They measured an increase in the number of large surface cells, indicating a reduced exfoliation rate, possibly due to the relatively stagnant post-lens tear film and the dampening effect of the lens on blink-mediated shear forces of the eyelid. Retained desiccated mucus, coarse mucous plaques, and palisading of cells also were observed. The authors suggested that tear film changes during overnight wear may result in increased epithelial permeability, leading to increased epithelial dehydration. Additionally, mature cells have fewer microvilli and less mucin and, according to Tsubota and Yamada (1992), thus may provide sites for bacterial adherence. In their study, Tsubota and Yamada (1992) found an increase in the mean cell area of the superficial corneal epithelium after 3 months' wear of disposable and conventional hydrogel lenses.

In a subsequent study, Tsubota et al. (1996) demonstrated that corneal epithelial cell size increases linearly with increasing overnight wear schedule and overall duration of hydrogel lens extended wear. After 6 months' wear, the mean epithelial cell area was significantly increased compared to baseline for subjects on a 3- or 6-nights-per-week extended-wear schedule, but not for subjects on a daily wear or 1 night per week extended-wear schedule. The investigators suggested that hypoxia delays apoptosis, or programmed cell death, leading to the retention of superficial cells.

Small crystallinelike deposits embedded in the superficial cornea have been identified during hydrogel lens extended wear (Bourassa and Benjamin 1988). Termed *microdeposits*, their composition, etiology, and clinical significance are unknown. Because these microdeposits are dislodged during lens removal or blinking after lens removal, regular lens removal was suggested as a means of limiting the impact of such microdeposits on the epithelium. Lin and Mandell (1991) also reported "corneal blotting" immediately on eye opening after overnight hydrogel lens wear. This type of lesion had a larger diameter and duller fluorescence than does punctate staining and typically corresponded to the position of back surface debris. It was suggested that "corneal blotting" represents an increase in epithelial permeability to fluorescein caused by an alteration in the mucin layer, and that therefore it has clinical significance with respect to the barrier function of the epithelium.

Epithelial Thickness

In most tissues, swelling occurs during oxygen deprivation. Yet even in the absence of oxygen (anoxia) for up to 6 hours, the corneal epithelium does not swell (O'Leary et al. 1981). Subjective reports of halos at the end of this period of exposure suggest, however, that changes occur in the intercellular spaces of the epithelium during anoxia.

Holden et al. (1985a) examined the clinical features of long-term unilateral hydrogel extended-wear lens wearers and measured a 5.6% reduction in corneal epithelial thickness in the lens-wearing eye. The epithelium required 7 days' cessation of lens wear to recover (see Figure 6.1). This finding has been verified by several investigators who used animal models of overnight hydrogel lens wear. In the monkey, Bergmanson et al. (1985) noted epithelial thinning without epithelial edema, as superficial cells were lost and the remaining cells were flattened. Madigan (1989) documented the effects of continuous lens wear by using monkey and cat models. Basal cell flattening and a decrease in the number and thickness of epithelial layers were noted. This structural compromise was linked with the altered metabolism and reduced mitosis accompanying chronic hypoxia.

The effects of short- or long-term conventional-lens versus disposable-lens extended wear on epithelial thickness are yet to be investigated. The statistical analysis of variables collected by Holden et al. (1985a) and noted earlier also found, however, that less epithelial thinning was associated with thinner lenses, more mobile lenses, and lenses that were replaced more frequently and removed more frequently. Individual characteristics that lessened the response were younger age, thinner corneas, and less polymegathous endothelium before commencing lens wear.

Microcysts

Intraepithelial cysts, or microcysts, are a useful and reliable clinical indicator of corneal hypoxic compromise during extended wear. Small numbers of microcysts have been observed also in asymptomatic non–contact lens wearers (Holden and Sweeney 1991). Microcysts are small (15–50 μm) and spherical or irregular in shape and are observed most frequently in the corneal midperiphery (Zantos and Holden 1978; Zantos 1981) (Figure 6.5). They move forward through the epithelium, reach-

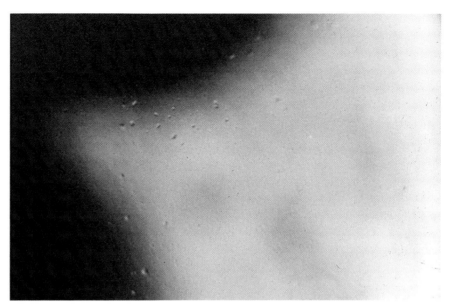

Figure 6.5 Slit-lamp photograph of corneal epithelial microcysts in a patient wearing hydrogel lenses on an extended-wear schedule. Microcysts are visible by using indirect illumination and high magnification, and display reversed illumination (i.e., the distribution of light within the microcysts is opposite to that of the background). (Photograph by Timothy Grant. Reprinted with permission from HA Swarbrick, BA Holden. Complications of Hydrogel Extended Wear. In JA Silbert [ed], Anterior Segment Complications of Contact Lens Wear. New York: Churchill Livingstone, 1994.)

ing significant numbers after approximately 2–3 months of extended hydrogel lens wear. After cessation of lens wear, the microcysts increase in number before disappearing within 2–3 months. Interestingly, Epstein and Donnenfeld (1989) and Efron and Veys (1992) reported the development of microcysts after relatively short periods of disposable-lens wear.

Typically, patients with microcysts are asymptomatic; the microcysts appear to cause no visual or other consequences. There is no apparent causal association between microcyst numbers and adverse inflammatory or infectious responses during extended wear of hydrogel lenses (Holden and Sweeney 1991). Holden et al. (1985b) were unable to identify an association between microcysts and any other clinical variables examined. However, Kenyon et al. (1986) noted subepithelial infiltrates in two patients who exhibited a concurrent severe microcyst response.

Zantos (1981) and Kenyon et al. (1986) proposed that the primary etiology for microcysts is hypoxic in nature, although this does not explain their midperipheral location. Other factors that may contribute include midperipheral lens bearing and chronic epithelial trauma (Zantos 1981, 1983). Josephson and Caffery (1979) suggest that cell death due to osmotic imbalance or the accumulation of debris and metabolic by-products in the post-lens tear film may stimulate the microcyst response. According to Epstein and Donnenfeld (1989), inadequate lens movement also may be a factor.

Based on the time course and clinical and histologic appearance of microcysts, Zantos (1983) believes that they are pockets of cellular debris, whereas Humphreys and Larke (1980) and Bergmanson (1987) suggest a dystrophic change or degeneration of epithelial cells. However, other possibilities, such as disorganized or incomplete cellular growth, fundamental changes in tissue synthesis, altered RNA, and ingested or phagocytosed necrotic tissue, have not been discounted. A suitable animal model for studying the microcyst response has yet to be identified because microcysts are not observed in either the monkey or the cat corneal epithelium with hypoxic stress (Madigan 1989). The availability of such a model would allow a better understanding of the cause and physiologic nature of microcysts.

The proposed hypoxic mechanism for the development of microcysts involves a reduction in epithelial mitotic rate and an increase in the regeneration time of the epithelium. Impaired cellular synthesis and waste removal are features related to altered metabolism. The increase in microcyst numbers after lens removal may be related to the return to normal epithelial metabolism and mitotic rate and subsequent accelerated removal of encapsulated cellular matter (Holden et al. 1985a).

Grant et al. (1987) reported a lower incidence of microcysts with extended wear of a high-water-content hydrogel lens, compared with a low-water-content hydrogel lens of the same oxygen transmissibility. The investigators speculated that greater peripheral oxygen was provided by the higher-water-content lens via diffusion and greater lens movement. According to Holden and Sweeney (1991), the microcyst response for rigid gas-permeable lenses is lower than that for hydrogel lenses of similar oxygen transmissibility. Characteristics of hydrogel lenses that may contribute to this finding include the reduced tear pump, complete corneal and limbal coverage, and greater pressure. These characteristics are similar for conventional and disposable extended-wear lenses with acceptable fitting characteristics.

Microcysts are primarily a function of reduced corneal oxygen supply, so it is not surprising that the number of microcysts is unaffected by regular lens replacement (Kotow et al. 1987a). Grant et al. (1988a, 1990) reported that disposable extended-wear lenses induce a microcyst response nearly identical to that of conventional extended-wear lenses. This study demonstrated that the number of microcysts increases with the number of consecutive nights of disposable-lens wear. In two other studies, however, the results were opposite: Poggio and Abelson (1993) noted a lower incidence of microcysts with disposable extended-wear lenses as compared with conventional extended-wear lenses in a multipractice retrospective study, whereas Epstein and Donnenfeld (1989) reported a higher incidence with disposable extended-wear lenses. Thus, this subject remains open to further study and interpretation.

Vacuoles

Vacuoles are another corneal intraepithelial cystic formation occurring during lens wear, and they have been noted also in small numbers in non–lens wearers. Typically, these formations are found in the presence of microcysts (Figure 6.6). Vacuoles are 20–50 μm in diameter, round, and located in the corneal midperiphery, sometimes in clusters (Zantos 1981). They display unreversed illumination and therefore are presumed to be gas- or fluid-filled epithelial spaces.

Vacuoles increase in numbers during extended wear (Holden et al. 1985b), but in contrast to microcysts, there is no increase in the number of vacuoles after cessation of lens wear (Grant et al. 1990). A link with corneal hypoxia has been presumed, owing to the time course of induction of vacuoles during lens wear. Their presence is considered to be relatively innocuous in terms of visual or other consequences.

Kotow et al. (1987a) reported that regular lens replacement does not decrease the number of vacuoles induced by extended wear. Grant et al. have studied extended wear of disposable and conventional lenses and noted a similar vacuole response in patients with both lens types (unpublished data).

Figure 6.6 Slit-lamp photograph of epithelial vacuoles in a patient wearing hydrogel lenses on an extended-wear schedule. Vacuoles are visible by using indirect illumination and high magnification, and display unreversed illumination (i.e., the distribution of light within the vacuoles is the same as that of the background).

Stroma

Corneal stromal changes induced by hydrogel extended-wear lenses may be due to structural, metabolic, and functional changes within the corneal epithelium; to a direct influence on the stroma itself; or to some combination of the two. Evidence for direct stromal effects exists from in vitro studies by Huff (1990), which demonstrated similar stromal edema levels with and without the epithelium in place. Huff (1990) also demonstrated that the stromal contribution to in vitro lens-induced edema was significant and dependent on stromal metabolism.

Stromal Thickness

Stromal swelling is a valuable clinical indicator of the state of corneal physiology. With extended wear of hydrogel lenses, increases in stromal thickness are significantly less in the periphery than in the center of the cornea, particularly in the presence of high levels of swelling (Mandell 1975; Bonanno and Polse 1985). Anoxia induced by goggles also produces the same differential response, demonstrating that tear exchange beneath the lens periphery is not a major factor in stromal swelling (Mandell 1975). It is likely that proximity to the more rigid sclera limits the swelling capability of the peripheral cornea.

   Both stromal edema and a 4.8% reduction in stromal thickness, with no evidence of structural abnormality, were recorded in long-term hydrogel lens extended wearers (Holden et al. 1985a). Immediately after lens removal, the stromal thinning was masked by marked edema; thinning became apparent only after 2 days' cessation of

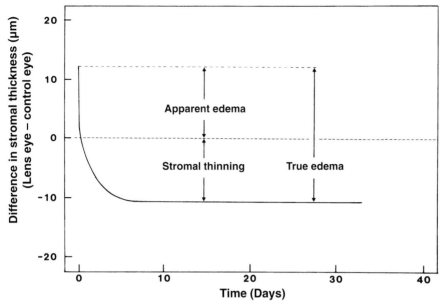

Figure 6.7 Decrease in stromal thickness of the long-term extended hydrogel lens–wearing eye after ceasing lens wear, indicating true edema, apparent edema, and stromal thinning. The dashed line at zero on the y axis represents the control eye data. (Reprinted with permission from BA Holden, DF Sweeney, A Vannas, et al. Effects of long-term extended contact lens wear on the human cornea. Invest Ophthalmol Vis Sci 1985;26:1489.)

lens wear (Figure 6.7). Less stromal thinning was associated with a thinner stroma, lower epithelial oxygen uptake rate, and less endothelial polymegathism before lens wear. Unlike the recovery of the epithelium, stromal recovery from chronic edema is slow. Stromal thinning has been reported up to 6 months after cessation of lens wear (Holden et al. 1985b).

On the basis of work by Kanai and Kaufman (1973), Bergmanson and Chu (1982), and Hart (1982), it has been suggested that chronic edema induces morphologic changes in stromal keratocytes, manifesting as functional changes in their ability to synthesize collagen, glycoproteins, and proteoglycans (Holden et al. 1985a). Another possibility is dissolution of stromal tissue, perhaps due to the effects of lactic acid on the stromal mucopolysaccharide ground substance. A relationship between corneal edema and loss of stromal glycosaminoglycans and proteoglycans has been identified in rabbit model studies by several investigators. Kangas et al. (1990) found that some glycosaminoglycans were lost within 3 hours of the onset of edema. Edema was demonstrated also to induce amino acids in an in vitro study by Kaye et al. (1982). The effect of these amino acids on the structure and function of glycosaminoglycans has yet to be determined. No data are available comparing the effects of conventional and disposable extended-wear lenses on stromal thickness during long-term lens wear.

Striae and Folds

Posterior stromal striae, first observed by Sarver (1971), indicate an acute change in corneal thickness. Striae are fine, gray-white lines that can be vertical, horizontal, or oblique. They are confined to the posterior third of the stroma and manifest as a

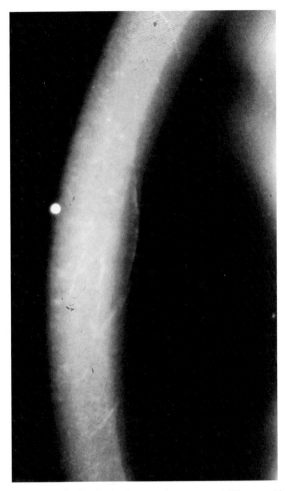

Figure 6.8 Slit-lamp photograph of striae in the posterior cornea, visible on waking from overnight hydrogel lens wear. (Reprinted with permission from SG Zantos, BA Holden. Ocular changes associated with continuous wear of contact lenses. Aust J Optom 1978;61:418.)

result of fluid separation of collagen fibrils (Figure 6.8). Striae are reversible and are not observed in all individuals after the same stimulus (Zantos 1981). The average critical levels of stromal swelling for the appearance of striae are 4.5% and 3.8% for vertical and horizontal striae, respectively (Zantos 1981).

Folds, appearing as black lines in the posterior stroma, are observed if 10–15% stromal swelling is present. Folds represent a physical buckling of the posterior stromal layers and Descemet's membrane. Klyce and Bernegger (1978) hypothesized that the buckling is caused by the shorter chord length of the posterior stromal lamellae and the restriction to swelling imposed by the scleral ring.

Striae and folds that appear during overnight hydrogel lens wear are a function of the oxygen transmissibility of the lens and the oxygen uptake rate of the cornea. Therefore, disposable and conventional lenses of similar oxygen transmissibilities will induce striae and folds to the same extent in the same cornea. Support for this reasoning is provided by Kotow et al. (1987a), who found that the degree of corneal swelling was unaffected by regular replacement of conventional lenses.

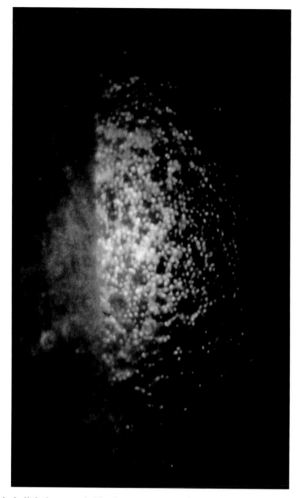

Figure 6.9 Endothelial photograph 20 minutes after hydrogel lens insertion in an unadapted subject. Blebs are irregular nonreflecting (black) areas within the endothelial mosaic. (Photograph by Steve Zantos and Brien Holden. Reprinted with permission from HA Swarbrick, BA Holden. Complications of Hydrogel Extended Wear. In JA Silbert [ed], Anterior Segment Complications of Contact Lens Wear. New York: Churchill Livingstone, 1994.)

Endothelium

Blebs

Blebs are a rapid, reversible change in the appearance of the corneal endothelial mosaic (Figure 6.9). Blebs manifest as areas of loss of reflectivity that gradually increase in size and appear slightly raised (Zantos and Holden 1977a). Vannas et al. (1984) demonstrated that blebs result from endothelial cell swelling and subsequent changes in the contours of cell membranes.

Zantos (1981) reported that this short-term response occurs with lens-induced hypoxia and atmospheric anoxia but not during silicone elastomer lens wear. The author proposed that blebs are caused by hypoxia and other changes in the cellular environ-

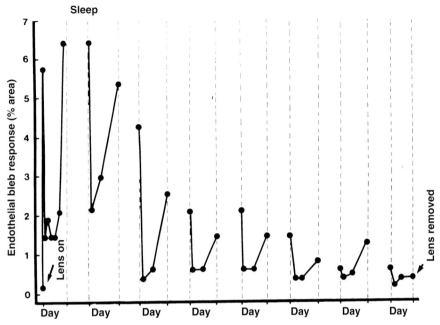

Figure 6.10 Typical endothelial bleb response in an unadapted subject over 7 days of continuous hydrogel lens wear. (Reprinted with permission from L Williams, BA Holden. The bleb response of the endothelium decreases with extended wear of contact lenses. Clin Exp Optom 1986;69:90.)

ment (and perhaps also by neurologic factors) because of the rapidity of the response. A reduced bleb response was observed in aphakic eyes after unilateral cataract surgery, further indicating a multifactorial etiology (Holden et al. 1982). Holden et al. (1985c) found that exposure to increased levels of carbon dioxide without the induction of corneal swelling also induced blebs. These investigators suggested that blebs are induced by decreased stromal pH, associated with both hypoxia and hypercapnia.

Zantos and Holden (1977a) and Vannas et al. (1981) measured the bleb response after lens insertion and recorded a maximum after approximately 30 minutes. With extended wear, there is a second peak in bleb numbers in the afternoon and evening of the second day and no detectable response after 6 days of continuous lens wear (Williams and Holden 1986) (Figure 6.10).

The bleb response occurs at precorneal oxygen levels below 15% (Williams 1986). Hence, blebs are observed to a similar extent with conventional and disposable hydrogel extended-wear lenses of similar oxygen transmissibility.

Polymegathism

Endothelial polymegathism, or increased variation in cell size, is a long-term morphologic change in the endothelial mosaic (Figure 6.11). Typically, it is accompanied by endothelial pleomorphism, characterized by a decrease in the frequency of hexagonal cells. Although Holden et al. (1985a) and others have measured no concurrent change in endothelial cell density during hydrogel lens wear, MacRae et al. (1986) hypothesized that polymegathism and pleomorphism precede reduced cell density because all three features were observed in long-term wearers. They subsequently reported an association between reduced endothelial cell density (<2,000 cells/mm^2) and signifi-

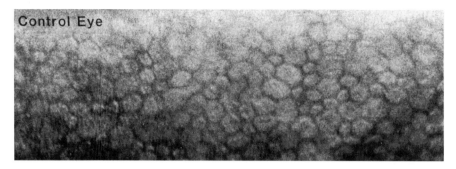

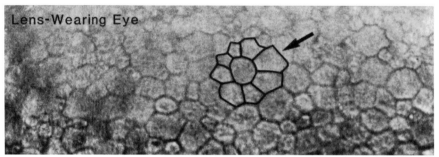

Figure 6.11 Endothelial photograph of non–lens-wearing control eye (top) and lens-wearing eye (bottom) of a subject who had worn a hydrogel lens in one eye only on an extended-wear basis for 79 months. A greater variation in endothelial cell size (polymegathism) is evident in the lens-wearing eye (original magnification ×370). (Reprinted with permission from BA Holden, DF Sweeney, A Vannas, et al. Effects of long-term extended contact lens wear on the human cornea. Invest Ophthalmol Vis Sci 1985;26:1489.)

cantly greater endothelial polymegathism (>0.60) and pleomorphism (frequency of hexagons, <40%) in 10% of long-term hard lens wearers (MacRae et al. 1994).

Polymegathism has been observed and quantified with daily and extended hydrogel, rigid gas-permeable, and hard lens wear and with increasing patient age. Generally, it is believed that polymegathism is not reversible on cessation of lens wear. Recently, however, a trend toward reduced polymegathism after up to 5 years' cessation of lens wear was reported (Sibug et al. 1991).

An extensive examination of patients who had worn hydrogel lenses on an extended-wear basis unilaterally over a long period found no association between polymegathism and other ocular characteristics (Holden et al. 1985a). The authors suggested a degree of functional interrelation between the epithelium and endothelium, however. Indeed, endothelial function is altered by a variety of stimuli, including changes in precorneal oxygen tension, temperature, osmolarity, electrolyte concentration, and metabolic inhibitors (Mishima et al. 1969).

The mechanism of polymegathism has yet to be explained fully. Also unknown at the time of this writing are the precise effects of these structural alterations on the functional integrity of the endothelium. Connor and Zagrod (1986) theorized that the cause of polymegathism involves a hypoxia-induced reduction in adenosine triphosphate (ATP) levels and changes in the concentrations of extracellular and intracellular calcium. In contrast, Stefansson et al. (1987) and Bonnano and Polse (1987a) advocated corneal acidosis as an etiologic factor.

Evidence for the roles of hypoxia and corneal acidosis was provided by Schoessler and Orsborn (1987) in a report of unilateral polymegathism in a patient with long-standing unilateral ptosis. Further, Schoessler et al. (1984) and others have noted that polymegathism does not occur as a result of silicone elastomer lens wear.

The possible risks associated with polymegathism are thought to include greater postoperative complications and uncontrollable corneal edema with aging (Rao et al. 1984; MacRae et al. 1989). Slow corneal deswelling (loss of functional reserve) has been associated with polymegathism in both the young and elderly in studies by O'Neal et al. (1984) and O'Neal and Polse (1986). Further functional impairment was demonstrated when increased endothelial permeability and increased endothelial pump rate were recorded for hydrogel lens extended-wear–induced polymegathous corneas (Dutt et al. 1989). This finding is in agreement with the observation of functional abnormalities in other conditions exhibiting endothelial morphologic changes, such as Fuchs' endothelial dystrophy. Additionally, polymegathism is one of the features of the corneal exhaustion or fatigue syndrome, as described by Pence (1988) and Sweeney (1992). This syndrome is thought to represent endothelial dysfunction brought on by chronic lens-induced hypoxia and acidosis.

There is some dispute as to whether the morphologic changes in the endothelium are a result of changes in cell size or of redistribution of cell mass, as suggested by Bergmanson (1990, 1992). Whatever the cause, it is a fact that an irregular mosaic is inherently unstable; thus, the barrier function of the endothelium would best be maintained by adjacent cells with similar dimensions (Rao et al. 1984).

Holden et al. (1985d) reported an increase in polymegathism within 2 weeks of hydrogel lens extended wear, indicating rapid morphologic change. The degree of polymegathism has been correlated with length of lens wear and degree of hypoxia by many investigators. In contrast, Yamaguchi et al. (1993) reported that the most significant change occurred in the first 3 months of lens wear, followed by stabilization over the next 9 months. Another investigation (MacRae et al. 1990) found no significant difference in polymegathism after 1 year of daily or extended hydrogel lens wear.

Regular lens replacement during extended wear has no effect on the degree of polymegathism (Kotow et al. 1987a). A clinical evaluation of disposable lenses for daily wear, intermittent extended wear, and extended wear by Grant and coworkers at our institution revealed that the increase in polymegathism was greatest in the extended-wear groups and that this increase was similar in extent to that found in conventional-lens extended-wear groups (unpublished data).

Limbus

Vascularization

Nutritional, inflammatory, mechanical, traumatic, and toxic stimuli can promote vessel penetration into the normally avascular cornea (Figure 6.12). During lens wear, particularly overnight wear, one or all of these stimuli may be present. An oxygen deficit exists, providing the nutritional stimulus. Lens deposits, back-surface debris, and inflammatory cell entrapment provide inflammatory and possibly toxic stimuli. Superficial epithelial trauma associated with lens dehydration, lens bearing, chronic limbal irritation during lens movement, damage during lens manipulation, and foreign body damage could provide traumatic stimuli.

Both daily and extended contact lens wear have been associated with corneal vascularization, and many investigators have undertaken to model the process. More than 45 years ago, Cogan (1949) proposed that loss of limbal tissue compactness

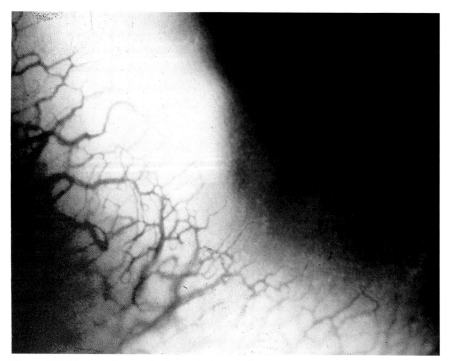

Figure 6.12 Slit-lamp photograph of vascularization of the peripheral cornea and limbal hyper-emia during hydrogel lens wear.

due to edema (stromal softening) was the stimulus to vessel growth. In 1980, Tomlinson and Haas reported that hydrogel lens–induced corneal edema of greater than 6% produced delayed vessel dilation and increased blood flow, lending support to Cogan's theory. Previous studies showed that stromal edema alone was an insufficient stimulus for vessel growth (Maurice et al. 1966), however. Holden et al. (1985e) also suggest that the reduced swelling response of the peripheral cornea, compared with that of the central cornea, implies that peripheral edema is not a significant factor promoting vascularization during hydrogel lens wear.

Several investigators have suggested some form of chemical mediator in corneal vascularization. Initially it was proposed that vasostimulatory factors neutralized growth-inhibiting substances (Maurice et al. 1966). Others since have advocated changes in positive chemotactic factors, including collagenases, proteases from inflammatory cells (Fromer and Klintworth 1976; Sholley et al. 1978), and secretions from damaged epithelial cells (Eliason 1978). Klintworth and Burger (1983) further suggested the involvement of locally generated or introduced vasoproliferative factors, in particular the cellular and humoral components of the inflammatory response, such as leukocytes, platelets, prostaglandins, plasminogen activator, and fibrin.

Plasminogen activator also has been implicated in the process of corneal vascularization by Berman et al. (1982). Support for this theory was provided by van Setten et al. (1990), who demonstrated an association between tear film plasmin levels and vascularization and reported increased tear plasmin concentrations during hydrogel lens extended wear, compared with other modalities of lens wear.

Hypoxia-related lactic acid accumulation within the cornea, in conjunction with reduced tissue compactness, also could provide the stimulus for vessel growth (Imre 1972). Work by Knighton et al. (1983) and Jensen et al. (1986) supports the theory of oxygen- and lactate-regulated angiogenic factors secreted by macrophages. Efron (1987) proposed a model for corneal vascularization in which hypoxia and epithelial damage are the initiating factors.

In an animal model of conventional hydrogel lens extended wear, Madigan et al. (1990) proposed a role for leukocytes and stromal keratocytes because of their close association with new vessels and absence during vessel regression. Rabbit model studies also suggested a relationship between corneal denervation and reduced vascularization and provided support for a neural control theory based on contact lens–induced neurologic deficits (Cassel and Groden 1984).

Limbal vessel dilation has been identified as the initial step in corneal vascularization. Chronic limbal vessel dilation would provide an active vascular plexus adjacent to the cornea on which stimuli promoting vessel growth could act. Limbal vessel engorgement is a common finding among hydrogel lens wearers (Zantos 1981). A study of unilateral long-term extended-wear hydrogel lens wearers demonstrated increased conjunctival and limbal hyperemia and vascularization in the lens-wearing eye compared with the nonwearing eye (Holden et al. 1986b). Two to 7 days after lens removal, the hyperemia was reduced significantly, but only insignificant vessel regression occurred after up to 33 days' cessation of lens wear.

Holden (1988) reported greater bulbar conjunctival redness in hydrogel lens extended-wear patients in comparison with non–lens wearers and those wearing hydrogel daily-wear lenses and rigid gas-permeable extended-wear lenses. More recently, Gauthier et al. (1992) found that long-term hydrogel lens wearers could be identified macroscopically on the basis of increased bulbar and limbal redness, compared with non–lens wearers and rigid gas-permeable lens wearers.

Although corneal vascularization has been reported during extended wear of both disposable and conventional lenses, quantitative data are rare. In one report on disposable-lens extended wear by Maguen et al. (1991), vascularization was associated only with a tightly fitting lens. This finding supports the suggestion that limbal compression and associated restricted venous outflow also are causal in vascularization. Nilsson and Lindh (1990) reported a low incidence of hyperemia with extended and flexible (occasional overnight) wear of disposable lenses. In a comparison of disposable-lens and conventional-lens extended wear in fellow eyes, Josephson et al. (1990) found no statistical difference in limbal response, although there appeared to be a trend toward reduced vascular response with regular lens replacement. These findings are in agreement with clinical studies conducted at our institution (unpublished data).

Because hypoxia is believed to be one of the major causal factors for vascularization, the extent of corneal vascularization with conventional and disposable lenses of similar oxygen transmissibility would be expected to be similar, with a trend toward a reduction with disposable extended-wear lenses resulting from reduced inflammatory stimuli and less irritation from lens deposits. New lens materials with high oxygen transmissibility are the most promising development for reducing the stimuli for vessel dilation and growth.

INFLAMMATION

Biocompatibility

Biocompatibility of a lens with the ocular surface includes both physical and chemical compatibility. Physical compatibility implies minimal or absent pressure, friction, or mechanical trauma to the ocular surface. Chemical compatibility generally relates to the absence—on the lens surface and in the polymer matrix—of deposition of tear film constituents and chemicals from lens care solutions. Factors that affect the extent of deposition include the lens surface and polymer chemistry, the patient's tear film composition, the lens care system, and the extent of denaturation of proteins already adherent to the lens.

Deposition is recognized as a significant problem during extended wear in terms of patient comfort and vision. An association between deposits on hydrogel lenses and ocular inflammation, including papillary conjunctivitis, also has been documented (Ballow et al. 1987; Rapacz et al. 1988). Additionally, deposition on lenses is important in terms of antigenicity to bound tear components and exogenous compounds.

Conclusive evidence has yet to be provided for an association between lens deposition and bacterial attachment because conflicting results have been obtained concerning the extent of bacterial attachment to worn (deposited) and unworn hydrogel lenses (Dart and Badenoch 1986; DiGaetano et al. 1986; Stern and Zam 1986; Butrus et al. 1987; Duran et al. 1987; Slusher et al. 1987; Barr et al. 1988; Prause et al. 1988; Aswad et al. 1990).

Several investigators have assessed the time course and mechanisms of hydrogel lens deposition. A variety of methodologies have been used, including electrophoresis, histochemical staining, standard analytical chemical assays, electron microscopy, immunofluorescence microscopy using radiolabeled proteins, and video image analysis. It has been demonstrated that proteins, lipids, and mucin are adsorbed readily and quickly onto, and absorbed within, a hydrogel lens matrix once it is exposed to the tear film (Newton-Howes et al. 1989; Cheng et al. 1990; Leahy et al. 1990; Lin et al. 1991; Hart et al. 1993). No one has been able to define a quantitative relationship between either the amount or type of deposit and the induction of visual effects, discomfort, or adverse responses, however.

Theoretically, ionic high-water-content hydrogel lenses absorb a greater quantity of tear proteins than do nonionic low-water-content lenses because of their inherently larger pore size and charged nature. This finding has been confirmed both clinically and in vitro. Sack et al. (1987) and Newton-Howes et al. (1989) noted that protein accumulation within the matrix of hydrogel lenses is dependent on the contact lens material composition and also on the size and charge of the protein molecules (Figure 6.13). The quantity of deposited protein, however, is not the only factor when considering complications due to lens spoilation. The type or state of the deposited protein also is likely to be important (Grant et al. 1989).

Several studies specifically have investigated deposition on lenses used for disposable extended wear. Leahy et al. (1990) demonstrated increased adsorption of lysozyme by ACUVUE, an ionic mid-water-content hydrogel lens, in comparison with nonionic lenses, after only a few minutes of lens wear. Lin et al. (1991) quantified the protein accumulation for ACUVUE and nonionic low-water-content See-Quence lenses (Bausch & Lomb, Rochester, NY) and also found significantly greater lysozyme adsorption on ACUVUE lenses. Additionally, this study demonstrated different time courses of lysozyme deposition for the two lens types. Deposition continued to increase with increasing wearing time for ACUVUE lenses, whereas for SeeQuence lenses, deposition stabilized after 24 hours. For other proteins, however, the time course of deposition was similar for the two lens types. These investigators also found significant variation in deposition rates among individual wearers.

In contrast, Vansted et al. (1986) found that the frequency and type of clinically discernible deposits on disposable lenses during extended wear were similar to those for conventional lenses during extended wear. Similarly, Nilsson and Lindh (1990)

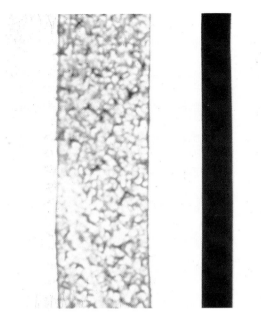

Figure 6.13 Photograph of sections of worn lenses stained for lysozyme. The right lens section is a SeeQuence lens (Bausch & Lomb, Rochester, NY) and the left lens section is an ACUVUE (Johnson & Johnson, Jacksonville, FL) lens. Both lenses had been worn on a daily-wear basis for 2 weeks. (Photograph by Nuria Durany, Cornea & Contact Lens Research Unit, University of New South Wales, Sydney, Australia.)

observed no clinical problems associated with lens deposition with either flexible (occasional overnight) or extended wear of ACUVUE lenses replaced every 2 weeks. At the same time, Josephson et al. (1990) reported their findings from a contralateral clinical trial of disposable- and conventional-lens extended wear. They found the surface appearance of 1-week-old ACUVUE lenses to be superior to that of 6-week-old conventional hydrogel lenses. These findings are in agreement with observations by Donshik et al. (1988) and clinical studies of conventional- and disposable-lens extended wear at our institution (unpublished data).

Because the material compositions of disposable and conventional lenses within the same United States Food and Drug Administration classification are essentially the same, the amount and type of deposition would be expected to be similar over periods involving the same duration and mode of lens wear. It is clear, however, that frequent lens replacement eliminates problems associated with lens aging and the accumulation and denaturation of deposits over time, such as lens discoloration, "jelly bumps" (raised, localized infiltrations of the lens matrix by tear film constituents, primarily calcium and protein), and lens calculi.

Contact Lens–Induced Papillary Conjunctivitis

Contact lens–induced papillary conjunctivitis is a chronic inflammatory response characterized by hyperemia, edema, and enlargement of papillae on the upper palpebral conjunctiva. Symptoms can include increased mucus secretion, itchiness, lens intolerance, blurred vision, and excessive lens movement, although in some cases the condition may be asymptomatic. Giant papillary conjunctivitis is a severe form of contact lens–induced papillary conjunctivitis, and this term also is applied to the disease when it is not associated with contact lens wear.

Clinical studies have demonstrated that the incidence of contact lens–induced papillary conjunctivitis is not related to the amount of protein within the lens matrix (Grant et al. 1989). An antigenic reaction to lens surface deposition, rather than to the lens material itself, was proposed as a mechanism for contact lens–induced papillary conjunctivitis by Allansmith et al. (1977). Support for an immunologic cause was further demonstrated in a clinical evaluation of unilateral lens replacement during hydrogel extended wear (Kotow et al. 1987a). The incidence of contact lens–induced papillary conjunctivitis was approximately 15% in both eyes, even though only one lens was replaced regularly.

There is evidence also to suggest a mechanical component in the development of papillary conjunctivitis because the reaction is induced also by ocular prostheses and protruding ocular sutures (Reynolds 1978; Srinivasan et al. 1979). Molinari (1983) theorized that, during lens wear, the antigens gain access to the mucous membrane as a result of chronic irritation of the conjunctiva by the lens edge or surface deposits. A degree of patient susceptibility also is believed to play a role (Fowler et al. 1979; Holden et al. 1986c). Duration of lens wear, lens age, and use of certain preserved solutions are other possible contributory factors (Fowler et al. 1979; Molinari 1983). A multifactorial etiology for papillary conjunctivitis during lens wear therefore is likely.

Extended wear of hydrogel lenses without regular replacement has been reported to cause contact lens–induced papillary conjunctivitis in approximately 50% of patients (Herman 1987; Grant et al. 1990), and regular lens replacement has been shown to reduce significantly the incidence of this problem (Holden et al. 1986c; Grant et al. 1988a, b; Ames and Cameron 1989; Boswall et al. 1993). In one retrospective study, however, the rate of occurrence of giant papillary conjunctivitis was similar for conventional- and disposable-lens extended wear (Poggio and Abelson 1993).

Further support for the advantages of regular lens replacement with respect to palpebral conjunctival inflammation can be found in the usefulness of disposable lenses on a daily or weekly disposal schedule for the management of patients with contact lens–induced papillary conjunctivitis (Grant et al. 1990; Marshall et al. 1992). Bucci et al. (1993), however, found no difference in palpebral response between conventional hydrogel lens–wearing eyes and monthly-replacement lens–wearing eyes in a 6-month contralateral evaluation with giant papillary conjunctivitis patients.

Tear-Borne Inflammatory Mediators and the Post-Lens Tear Film

A number of significant changes occur in the ocular environment during eye closure and are reversed rapidly after eye opening (Table 6.1). Baum (1990) and Sack et al. (1992) reported cessation or significant reduction of reflex tear secretion on eye closure. This manifests clinically as a reduced aqueous layer and more viscous tear film immediately on eye opening, as reported by Gilbard et al. (1988) and others.

The absence of blinking, of significant eye movements, and of tear flow during eye closure results in an accumulation of metabolic by-products, mucoprotein, exfoliated epithelial cells, and debris in the closed-eye tear film (Figure 6.14). Because hydrogel lenses frequently are immobile or adherent to the ocular surface on eye opening after sleep (Kenyon et al. 1988), the wearing of a contact lens during eye closure traps these components close to the corneal epithelium. Debris breakdown is thought to produce

Table 6.1 Ocular Environment in the Closed and Open Eye

Characteristic	Closed Eye	Open Eye	Study
Cornea			
pH	7.39	7.54	Bonanno and Polse 1987b
Temperature (°C)	36.2	34.5	Hill 1978
Tear film			
pH	7.25	7.45	Carney and Hill 1976
Tonicity (% NaCl)	0.89	0.97	Terry and Hill 1978
Oxygen (mm Hg)	61	155	Holden and Sweeney 1985
Carbon dioxide (mm Hg)	55	0	Holden et al. 1987

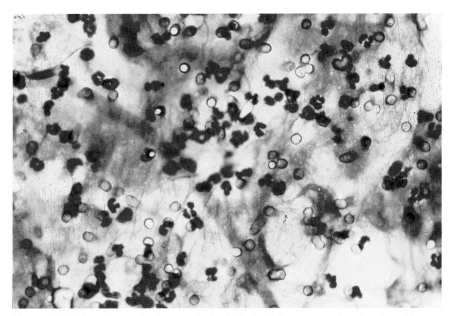

Figure 6.14 Light-microscopic photograph of cells isolated from a corneal wash collected by using the noncontact corneal irrigation technique immediately after sleep. Numerous epithelial cells, neutrophils (stained pink), and mucus strands are visible (original magnification ×900). (Photograph by Nicolette Sansey, Cornea & Contact Lens Research Unit, University of New South Wales, Sydney, Australia.)

substances toxic to the epithelium. This has been proposed as a mechanism for causing acute inflammatory reactions during extended wear (Zantos and Holden 1978; Mertz and Holden 1981). Yet to be determined are the critical levels and composition of post-lens tear film metabolic products and debris that could trigger such reactions.

Josephson et al. (1990) conducted a contralateral evaluation of disposable lenses and conventional nonreplaced lenses on an extended-wear schedule for 6 weeks. Of the 31 patients enrolled, two discontinued disposable-lens extended wear due to corneal staining associated with post-lens tear film debris. No patients discontinued conventional-lens extended wear for similar reasons. Lens-fitting characteristics, rather than the lens material itself, are likely to contribute to this finding.

Lens-fitting characteristics and the level of back-surface debris are unchanged by regular replacement of conventional lenses (Kotow et al. 1987a). There is some controversy as to the ability of lenses that are available in a limited number of combinations of base curves and diameters to exhibit sufficient lens movement to allow adequate post-lens tear exchange, which would reduce the contact time between inflammatory mediators and the corneal epithelium and limbal vasculature. It has been suggested that 0.2 mm of movement is adequate for hydrogel extended-wear lenses (Holden 1988). There are no published data comparing the extent of lens movement with conventional and disposable extended-wear lenses. Fitting studies at our institution have demonstrated, however, that a similar percentage of patients exhibit an acceptable lens fit and similar levels of lens movement with disposable and conventional lenses in standard parameters.

The proximity of the conjunctival and limbal vasculature to the cornea allows a rapid accumulation of circulating cellular and humoral components on appropriate stimulation. Josephson and Caffery (1979) suggested that infiltrates, which are thought to be composed primarily of leukocytes, may be derived also from the palpebral conjunctival vasculature. During eye closure without lens wear, there is a significant increase in the number of cells in the precorneal tear film (see Figure 6.14). In a study by Wilson et al. (1989), the median number of epithelial cells increased from 10 to 118 after 8 hours of sleep. The change was more dramatic and possibly of greater clinical significance for polymorphonuclear leukocytes, with their numbers increasing from 9 to 6,500 after sleep.

In an in vitro model developed by Elgebaly et al. (1985), leukocytes were observed to adhere to the superficial epithelial layer before penetrating beneath it. The infiltration occurred during exposure to what the investigators termed low levels of cells (10^5–10^7 cells/ml) for 5–60 minutes. Longer exposure times and higher numbers of cells led to deeper penetration and epithelial injury. This finding indicates that leukocytes have the capacity for causing corneal injury under certain conditions.

It has been proposed that leukocytes in the post-lens tear film during hydrogel lens extended wear are responsible for microabrasions, contact lens–induced acute red eye, and infiltrative keratitis (Josephson and Caffery 1989). Wilson et al. (1989) demonstrated that the leukocyte-to-epithelial cell ratio immediately on eye opening was increased by overnight wear of hydrogel lenses. In contrast, Fleiszig et al. (1992) found no difference between extended-wear hydrogel lens wearers and non–lens wearers in the number of precorneal leukocytes and bacteria attached to the leukocytes in the open eye. There are no comparative data for precorneal cell counts during disposable- and conventional-lens extended wear.

In recent years, there have been major advances in quantifying the biochemical components of the precorneal tear film. Contact lens wear has been shown to increase the concentration of plasmin in the tear film (Tervo et al. 1989; van Setten et al. 1990; Vannas et al. 1992). Plasmin inhibits wound healing and can break down fibrin to initiate the chemotaxis of leukocytes, particularly neutrophils. Tervo et al. (1990) also isolated plasmin in association with adherent bacteria on the surface of worn contact lenses.

The detection of complement in the tear film of normal subjects by Chandler et al. (1974) and several others also is an important finding. The primary role of complement is defensive. Many compounds can activate the complement cascade, the end point of which is tissue damage and inflammation. Activated complement is a potent leukotactic agent. Mondino et al. (1977, 1978) were the first to suggest that the activation of complement is involved in corneal inflammation.

Vitronectin also has been isolated in the precorneal tear film of normal eyes without lens wear, and the concentration was found to increase significantly during sleep (Sack et al. 1993). As an inhibitor of plasmin and complement-mediated damage, vitronectin may play a role in the maintenance of closed-eye corneal homeostasis.

A significant increase in tear film calcium and total protein with prolonged eye closure was first noted by Huth et al. (1981). Sack et al. (1992) also measured significant biochemical changes in the tear film during eye closure without lens wear. The major protein components of open-eye tear fluid are lysozyme, lactoferrin, and tear-specific prealbumin. With eye closure, secretory IgA and albumin become the major components, and both complement C3 and plasminogen are activated. In combination with the documented increase in precorneal polymorphonuclear leukocytes, these changes are indicative of a subclinical inflammatory state during sleep. Sack et al. (1992) believe that this environment represents a protective mechanism against pathogens entrapped in the closed eye because of the absence of blinking and tear flow. They also suggested, however, that inflammatory and immune-mediated pathologic reactions, such as those seen during overnight wear of hydrogel lenses, may be promoted in such an environment.

Further work has shown that the changes in tear film composition during sleep occur in a specific sequence (Tan et al. 1993). These authors suggest that activation of complement C3 within 1–3 hours of eye closure may promote the release of chemotactic factors that then induce a rapid accumulation of polymorphonuclear leukocytes after 3–5 hours of eye closure. They also suggest that inflammation and other adverse responses during overnight hydrogel lens wear may be the result of an alteration of one or more of the features of this sequence of events. A comparison of the effects of disposable- and conventional-lens extended wear on the components and sequence of events in the closed-eye tear film is yet to be conducted.

The biologic functions of other chemical and cellular mediators in the tear fluid and ocular tissue are being examined with respect to the modulation of corneal and other ocular inflammation. These include mediators of plasma origin, such as the kinin system and clotting system, and also mediators of tissue origin, such as vasoactive amines, the arachidonic cascade, lysozymal components, and lymphocyte products (Chiou and Chang 1990). The roles of cytokines, prostanoids, and growth factors in immune responses of the cornea also are under investigation (Kehrl et al. 1986; Ellingsworth et al. 1988; Shams et al. 1994). In vitro model studies are being conducted to increase understanding of these mediators, their receptors, signal transduction pathways, and mechanisms of regulation, with a long-term goal of developing sensitive therapeutic agents that act at a molecular level (Bazan and Bazan 1990).

In summary, the results of various studies indicate that a number of biologic components within the precorneal tear film and cornea are capable of inducing inflammation. The interactions between the host and these entities are complex. Extended wear offers the opportunity for increased and often chronic stimuli to inflammatory processes within the cornea, but the causes of these lens-induced events are not understood fully. It is possible that the unique anatomy, function, and immunology of the anterior ocular structures may have created a system in which inflammatory and immunologic mechanisms are also unique, lessening the relevance of knowledge gained through observation in other body tissues (Elgebaly et al. 1985).

Corneal Infiltrates

Corneal infiltrates represent an accumulation of cellular components of serum that have leaked from adjacent vessels in response to one or more stimuli (Figure 6.15). Both Hogan and Zimmerman (1962) and Marshall and Grindall (1978) reported the

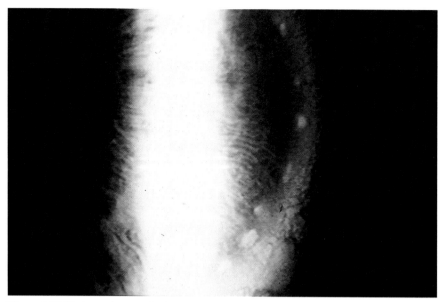

Figure 6.15 Slit-lamp photograph of peripheral corneal infiltrates during daily wear of disposable lenses. (Photograph by Robert Terry, Cornea & Contact Lens Research Unit, University of New South Wales, Sydney, Australia.)

presence of lymphocytes in the basal layer of the healthy human corneal epithelium, implying a normal baseline level of infiltration. Basu and Minta (1976) also demonstrated that polymorphonuclear leukocytes can move readily within the stroma, yet an intact epithelium and Descemet's membrane are barriers to their movement. Clinically, cellular aggregations have been observed within both the corneal stroma and the epithelium, in both symptomatic and asymptomatic individuals and with and without other ocular signs (Zantos and Holden 1977b; Josephson and Caffery, 1979). Typically, the cells are distributed diffusely or in foci or bands.

Several investigators consider infiltrates to be one of the most common adverse reactions during lens wear (Josephson and Caffery 1979; Zantos 1984; Gordon and Kracher 1985; Josephson et al. 1988). Infiltrates occur more frequently with hydrogel lens wear than with rigid gas-permeable lens wear (Josephson and Caffery 1979; Vajdic et al. 1995) and are more severe in hydrogel lens wearers than in non–lens wearers (Josephson and Caffery 1979). According to Dart (1986), corneal infiltrates similar to those occurring in association with staphylococcal blepharitis in non–lens wearers commonly are observed during hydrogel lens extended wear and may be caused by a reaction to antigens on the lens.

In the cornea, inflammatory cells are attracted chemotactically, mostly via the activation of complement, and they then can play a chemotactic role themselves (Jackson and Gilmore 1981). Cellular infiltration can occur extremely rapidly and is indicative of inflammation. Infiltrates have been reported to occur in response to tissue injury, hypoxia, toxins, bacteria, viruses, parasites, solution preservatives, other exogenous compounds, and immunoglobulins and as an idiopathic reaction. In some cases, it is difficult to determine the exact cause of infiltration or to distinguish between lens-related and other precipitating factors.

Using a rabbit model, Mondino et al. (1981) found that corneal infiltrates consist of polymorphonuclear leukocytes and mononuclear cells. Immature plasma cells also have been reported (Rietschel and Wilson 1982). Generally, it is agreed that viral stimuli induce migration of mononuclear cells, such as lymphocytes, and bacterial stimuli induce a polymorphonuclear leukocyte response, particularly neutrophils. Further, a lymphocytic response indicates a mild reaction, whereas a polymorphonuclear leukocyte response typically occurs in cases of severe acute inflammation (Leibowitz 1984).

On activation, neutrophils are capable of releasing cytotoxic products, including proteolytic enzymes, arachidonic acid metabolites, and active oxygen-derived species (Alio et al. 1993). These products, particularly the oxygen free-radical superoxide anion, cause tissue damage. Carubelli et al. (1990) demonstrated that oxygen radicals, in association with polymorphonuclear leukocytes, are active in inflammatory and ulcerative corneal lesions.

Leukotrienes are chemotactic for polymorphonuclear leukocytes, and molecules involved in their production, the lipoxygenases, are synthesized within the cornea (Samelsson 1980; Bazan and Bazan 1990). Components of the complement pathways also have been isolated within the cornea and later were shown to be concentrated in the peripheral cornea (Mondino et al. 1980). These investigators speculated that the source of complement components may include the limbal vasculature, the tear film, the aqueous humor, or the corneal cells themselves. Activation of these compounds could result in the release of potent chemotactic factors C3a and C5a, which may be responsible for the rapid nature of cellular infiltration into the cornea. Stromal keratocytes also are believed to play an active role in the corneal inflammatory response, possibly through their phagocytic capability (Henriquez 1987; Madigan 1989; Madigan et al. 1990).

Gordon and Kracher (1985) conducted a retrospective analysis of corneal infiltrates during conventional-lens extended wear by a population with a significant proportion of aphakic patients. This investigation revealed that the majority of infiltrates were located within 3 mm of the limbus (93%) and beneath the upper lid (67%). The authors suggested that the superior location was due to greater corneal hypoxia in that region. A tight lens fit and post-lens tear film debris also were associated with infiltrates. It is possible, however, that some of the events reported in this study were in fact corneal ulcers because overlying corneal staining was a feature in 44% of cases, the episodes were symptomatic, and some resulted in corneal scarring.

Theoretically, if lens deposition and the accumulation of back-surface debris are causative factors in corneal infiltration, one would predict a higher incidence with conventional nonreplaced hydrogel lenses as compared with disposable lenses. However, there have been no controlled clinical studies comparing the incidence of corneal infiltrates (without overlying epithelial disruption) during conventional- and disposable-lens extended wear, although anecdotal reports and some studies have suggested a higher incidence with disposable lenses. In a multipractice retrospective study, Poggio and Abelson (1993) suggested that the incidence of sterile peripheral infiltrates was higher with disposable-lens extended wear than with conventional-lens extended wear. Boswall et al. (1993) also noted a trend toward increased peripheral infiltration with disposable-lens compared with conventional-lens extended wear, although the trend was not statistically significant.

Baum and Barza (1990) proposed that frequent lens removal or replacement would not reduce the risk of corneal infiltrates. In a multicenter clinical evaluation of disposable lenses worn on a 6-night extended-wear basis, Port (1991) reported that sterile corneal infiltrates were observed in 1–9% of patients. Maguen et al. (1991, 1992, 1994) reported the results of a retrospective chart review of patients who wore disposable lenses for extended wear over a 3-year period. In the first year, among

100 patients, there were six cases of peripheral corneal infiltrates; in the second year, 13 patients were lost to follow-up, and there were seven cases of corneal infiltrates; in the third year, 23 additional patients were lost to follow-up, and one case of corneal infiltrate was recorded. It is noteworthy that these events, although classified as corneal infiltrates, were accompanied by a break in the overlying epithelium, which we would classify as infiltrative keratitis. Another interesting finding during a short-term study comparing defective versus nondefective disposable lenses was the occurrence of two cases of peripheral corneal infiltration within 6 hours of wearing lenses with edge defects (Efron and Veys 1992).

Recently, Suchecki et al. (1996) reported the results of a retrospective analysis of patients presenting to their practice with contact lens–associated peripheral corneal infiltrates with and without overlying epithelial involvement. The overlying staining ranged from superficial punctate keratitis to a frank epithelial defect. At the time of the event, 40% of patients were wearing disposable lenses on an extended-wear basis, and 21% were wearing conventional lenses on an extended-wear basis. The numbers of disposable-lens and conventional-lens extended wearers served by this practice are unknown, so this result is uninterpretable with respect to the effect of lens type. The authors developed an inflammatory index as a measure of the severity of the event and found no difference between events during disposable-lens and conventional-lens extended wear. Corneal bacterial cultures were performed for some patients, and there was no relationship between positive or negative cultures and lens type.

Cutter et al. (1996) conducted a large prospective cross-sectional multicenter study of focal corneal infiltrates with overlying fluorescein staining in hydrogel lens wearers. The overlying staining ranged from superficial stippling to a frank epithelial defect. The overall prevalence rate was found to be 1.6% (95% confidence interval [CI] 1.12–2.16) of patients examined. For all extended-wear lens wearers, current smoking was a significant risk factor (odds ratio [OR] 3.21, 95% CI 1.05–9.76). For daily- and extended-wear lens wearers, there was increased risk associated with disposable- compared with conventional-lens wear of 2.1 ($P = .036$). When only extended wear was considered, the risk for disposable-lens wear relative to conventional-lens wear was insignificant ($P = .236$). When smoking status was controlled for, however, the risk for disposable-lens extended wear relative to conventional-lens extended wear was significant (OR = 8.35, 95% CI 1.08–64.46).

In their interpretation of this finding, the authors suggested that a combination of factors was responsible, including the use of disposable lenses for longer periods compared with conventional lenses, a high proportion of ionic lens materials among the disposable-lens types, modified practitioner prescribing patterns for disposable lenses (i.e., poorer patient selection and education), modified patient attitudes and behaviors about disposable lenses, the differential ability of disposable- and conventional-lens wearers to appropriately self-manage after the onset of symptoms, and the recommendation by practitioners of "looser" lens care regimens with disposable lenses. These are important observations that should not be overlooked when comparing all aspects of disposable- and conventional-lens performance.

Well-controlled clinical trials with a substantial sample size are needed to determine the incidence of corneal infiltrates during conventional- and disposable-lens wear. In addition, ongoing biochemical and immunologic work is required to identify the stimuli that induce an influx of inflammatory cells into the cornea. These studies may enable the isolation and development of compounds that impede or inhibit specific inflammatory pathways, which subsequently may be incorporated into lenses, either conventional or disposable, or lens care systems.

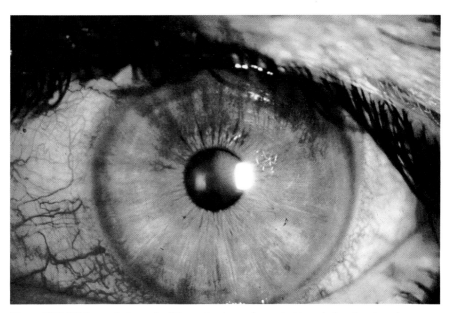

Figure 6.16 Slit-lamp photograph of the acute phase of a contact lens–induced acute red eye reaction during hydrogel lens extended wear. (Photograph by Timothy Grant. Reprinted with permission from HA Swarbrick, BA Holden. Complications of Hydrogel Extended Wear. In JA Silbert [ed], Anterior Segment Complications of Contact Lens Wear. New York: Churchill Livingstone, 1994.)

Contact Lens–Induced Acute Red Eye Reaction

Contact lens–induced acute red eye (CLARE) is an inflammatory reaction occurring subsequent to eye closure during lens wear. The patient experiences no symptoms before eye closure but is awakened from sleep by marked ocular discomfort or experiences slight to mild irritation or pain on eye opening. Redness, and in some cases watery discharge, swollen eyelids, and photophobia, are characteristic clinical features (Zantos and Holden 1978). Clinical signs include bulbar conjunctival and limbal blood vessel engorgement, multiple midperipheral subepithelial or stromal infiltrates, occasional minor corneal staining, and a mild anterior chamber reaction in severe cases (Figure 6.16).

Contact lens–induced acute red eye reaction is overwhelmingly a hydrogel lens–related phenomenon, although it has been reported in association with persistent rigid gas-permeable lens adherence following overnight wear (Schnider et al. 1988). In clinical studies at our institution, contact lens–induced acute red eye has been observed only during rigid gas-permeable lens extended wear in patients who previously had experienced one or more episodes during hydrogel lens extended wear.

Sweeney et al. (1993) reported that the majority of contact lens–induced acute red eye cases observed in a series of clinical studies (83%, $n = 88$) were monocular, with no predilection for a particular eye. The lens-wearing time before the first episode was variable, ranging from 0.1 to 42 months (mean, 23 ± 24 months; Sweeney et al. 1993). A patient can experience the problem on more than one occasion if extended wear is continued. In this situation, the probability is 56% for a second reaction and 47% for a third event. The wearing time before second and third events is variable, and the reaction can occur in the same or in the contralateral eye.

The finding of subsequent episodes during either hydrogel or rigid gas-permeable lens wear suggests some degree of patient sensitization after the first event.

The exact mechanism of contact lens–induced acute red eye is not fully understood, although several hypotheses have been advanced. Hodd (1977) proposed that the reaction occurs when lenses are not removed frequently enough for cleaning. Zantos and Holden (1978) suggested an immunologic cause associated with an accumulation of debris and toxins on or beneath the lens. Mertz and Holden (1981) isolated mucus, squamous epithelial cell remnants, and neutrophils in the post-lens debris from an individual experiencing contact lens–induced acute red eye, and proposed that this combination of substances, when trapped beneath an immobile lens, is capable of stimulating the inflammatory response.

Phillips (1979) hypothesized a multifactorial etiology, including the suppression of epithelial regeneration due to anoxia or poor lens fitting, a conjunctivitis-like reaction caused by pathogens trapped by mucus adhesion, and such patient factors as intense emotional strain. Zantos (1984) examined several variables and found no association with patient age, sex, refractive error, history, season, or length of lens wear. Hypoxia is unlikely to be a major factor, because a contact lens–induced acute red eye reaction has been documented at our institution with overnight wear of a bound silicone elastomer lens.

Bacterial contamination has been implicated by several investigators as a causal factor in contact lens–induced acute red eye. The organisms themselves or toxins released by these organisms may stimulate the response. A toxin-related response also was suggested by Phillips et al. (1986), who noted that this reaction typically occurs soon after reuse of cleaned and disinfected conventional lenses, when endotoxin from nonviable bacteria may be present. Dohlman et al. (1973) reported the isolation of *Staphylococcus aureus* from five of seven patients who experienced an inflammatory reaction suggestive of contact lens–induced acute red eye during therapeutic continuous wear.

Work at our institution shows that individuals who experience contact lens–induced acute red eye reaction have a higher incidence of gram-negative bacterial contamination of their lenses than wearers who have never had this reaction (Baleriola-Lucas et al. 1991). This finding, in combination with changes that occur in the ocular environment during overnight wear, is under further investigation. Further support for a bacterial cause (Holden et al. 1996) is provided by a study in which the overnight wear of hydrogel lenses inadvertently contaminated with gram-negative bacteria was found to trigger a contact lens–induced red eye reaction in 33% of subjects and corneal infiltrates in an additional 42% of subjects.

Valuable insight into possible contributing factors has been provided by comparison of the incidence of contact lens–induced acute red eye reaction among different populations using different overnight wear modes, lens types, lens replacement frequencies, and care systems. During a continuous-wear study using conventional lenses, the incidence was 34% (Zantos and Holden 1978). The worst-case scenario appears to occur with conventional high-water-content hydrogel lenses subjected to heat disinfection. In one study, the incidence of contact lens–induced acute red eye over 1 year using this conventional lens type and heat disinfection was 56% (Kotow et al. 1987b).

Regular lens replacement significantly reduces the incidence of contact lens–induced acute red eye compared with yearly lens replacement (Rengstorff 1983; Crook 1985). In studies at our institution, regular lens replacement was found to reduce the incidence from 15% to 2% for low-water-content hydrogel lenses (Kotow et al. 1987a) and from 14% to 5% for high-water-content lenses (Grant et al. 1987). The lowest incidence was reported with replacement of low-water-content conventional lenses every 3 months, coupled with weekly removal for surfactant cleaning, peroxide disinfection, and enzymatic cleaning (Kotow et al. 1987b).

Insufficient lens movement has been suggested also as a contributing factor (Nilsson and Lindh 1990). Hence, single-parameter disposable lenses may carry a greater risk. No cases of contact lens–induced acute red eye were observed in disposable-lens extended-wear studies conducted by Gruber (1988), Ivins (1988), and Michielsen et al. (1990). In other disposable-lens studies, Donshik et al. (1988) reported one event in a 733-patient study, and Woods (1989) reported two events in a 41-patient study. In extended-wear lens studies at our institution, the incidence of contact lens–induced acute red eye was relatively low after 12 months of disposable-lens wear (6%) as compared with conventional-lens wear (15%) (Grant 1991). In a study of intermittent extended wear (two consecutive nights per week) of disposable lenses replaced on a monthly basis compared with daily wear, Grant et al. (1988a) observed no contact lens–induced acute red eye events in either group.

This acute, intense inflammatory reaction is of major significance to both patients and practitioners. The etiology is likely to be multifactorial and, at present, the most promising approach to finding the cause appears to be an investigation of bacterial contamination and corneal and tear-borne inflammatory mediators. Such research may allow the development of preventative measures or the identification of predisposed individuals before they commence overnight lens wear.

Contact Lens Peripheral Ulceration

As described here, contact lens peripheral ulcers are a phenomenon associated almost exclusively with hydrogel lens extended wear. Although the signs are unique, it is possible that some events may be misdiagnosed as infectious keratitis. Contact lens peripheral ulcers can manifest at any time of the day. The severity of irritation is variable, with the majority of patients reporting mild to moderate levels of discomfort in the form of scratchiness or foreign body sensation that increases in severity when the lens is removed (Sweeney et al. 1993). Other signs and symptoms may include localized or diffuse bulbar and limbal injection, watery discharge, swollen lids, and photophobia. Some patients are asymptomatic.

The typical lesion is circular, well defined, and located in the corneal periphery or midperiphery. A focal excavation of the epithelium and Bowman's membrane, stromal disorganization, and underlying and surrounding stromal infiltrates are present during the active stage. Occasionally, a concurrent, clinically significant microcyst response and endothelial bedewing (cells adherent to the central-inferior corneal endothelium) are observed. With cessation of lens wear, the acute reaction is self-limiting. The lesion resolves without medical intervention, leaving a circular subepithelial scar (Figure 6.17).

In clinical studies at our institution, this form of ulcer has not recurred in patients who have returned to extended lens wear after resolution of the lesion (Sweeney et al. 1993). The average lens-wearing time before a contact lens peripheral ulcer was seen in these studies was 39 ± 29 months, with a range from 4.5 to 67 months. Interestingly, these ulcers were found to occur more frequently in the right eye. One episode was observed during daily hydrogel lens wear. Contact lens peripheral ulcers, as described here, have not been reported in patients wearing hard or rigid gas-permeable lenses.

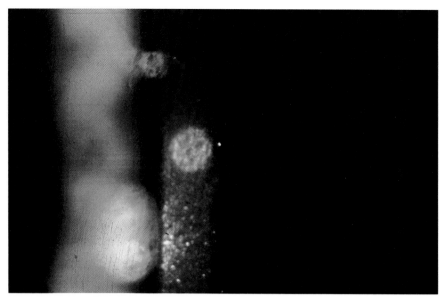

Figure 6.17 Slit-lamp photograph of the scar from a healed contact lens peripheral ulcer that developed during soft lens extended wear. (Photograph by Deborah Sweeney, Cornea & Contact Lens Research Unit, University of New South Wales, Sydney, Australia.)

The etiology of contact lens peripheral ulcers is unknown. Analysis of events during a series of clinical studies at our institution revealed no common factors among patient characteristics or lens-wearing histories (Sweeney et al. 1993). Several theories have been proposed, including hypersensitivity, toxic and immune reactions, and hypoxia-related factors. Endotoxin from gram-negative bacteria also has been implicated in the response. Catania (1987) contended, however, that endotoxin would induce widespread inflammation of the tissue. Unlike the ulcer described here, epithelial defects after exposure to endotoxin typically are large and central, involve deep stromal layers, and induce considerable corneal edema and a mucopurulent discharge.

Bates et al. (1989) suggested that sterile ulcers represent early or spontaneously resolving microbial episodes. The authors identified a significant relationship between sterile keratitis and both poor lens hygiene and lens case contamination by bacteria.

It has been hypothesized that peripheral ulcers and infiltrates that develop during lens wear are the result of hypersensitivity to certain components of bacteria, particularly staphylococci (Smolin et al. 1979). Peripheral, self-limiting ulceration has been reported in non–lens wearers in association with staphylococcal colonization of the adnexa (Chignell et al. 1970; Catania 1987). Typically, these lesions occur at the 4 and 8 o'clock positions. In contrast, contact lens peripheral ulcers have no predilection for these corneal positions. Further, patients with this type of ulcer seen at our institution have not had concurrent lid or conjunctival disease, unlike patients with catarrhal ulcers. The lack of recurrence and the well-defined, circular, nonprogressive features also suggest that contact lens peripheral ulcers are not related to bacterial hypersensitivity per se.

The microbiologic analysis of lenses recovered during an event do suggest, however, that gram-positive bacteria adherent to a contact lens are involved in the pathogenesis of these ulcers (Willcox et al. 1995). In this study, patients with high levels of gram-positive bacteria on their lenses at routine aftercare visits were significantly more likely to develop a contact lens peripheral ulcer than were noncarriers.

The nonprogressive nature of these ulcers may be related to peripheral corneal anatomy. There are more Langerhans' cells in the peripheral cornea than in the central cornea (Klareskog et al. 1979; Streilein et al. 1979; Bergstresser et al. 1980). According to van Klink et al. (1993), Langerhans' cells are efficient antigen-presenting cells and may accelerate protective immunity, as demonstrated in an in vitro study in which *Acanthamoeba* keratitis was inhibited by the induction of Langerhans' cells. Other investigations have demonstrated the opposite effect, however (McLeish et al. 1989; Jager et al. 1990).

Regular lens replacement does not reduce the incidence of contact lens peripheral ulcers (Grant et al. 1991). There also appears to be no significant difference in the incidence of these ulcers during conventional- and disposable-lens extended wear at our institution (2.9% versus 3.4% per patient year respectively; unpublished data). Many cases of sterile infiltrative keratitis have been reported during disposable-lens extended wear, however (Harris et al. 1989; Serdahl et al. 1989; Maguen et al. 1991; Matthews et al. 1992; Poggio and Abelson 1993). Shovlin (1989) reviewed some of the cases from the preceding studies and concluded that lack of lens movement was an important factor and that the typical patient was young, female, and a previous lens wearer.

In a retrospective study, Marshall et al. (1992) determined that the relative risk of developing noninfectious keratitis during disposable-lens extended wear was one-third the risk with conventional-lens extended wear. In contrast, in a report of a multipractice retrospective study of disposable-lens and conventional-lens extended wear, Poggio and Abelson (1993) suggested that there was a greater incidence of sterile peripheral keratitis with disposable lenses. The evidence is therefore inconclusive. It should be noted that between-study comparisons of the incidence of contact lens peripheral ulcers and other presumed or confirmed noninfectious keratitis events with various lens types and wear schedules are difficult because of differences in clinical definitions of this response among the various investigators.

CORNEAL INFECTION

Risk Factors for Infectious Keratitis

The annualized incidence of infectious keratitis is 21–34 per 10,000 overnight hydrogel lens wearers (Poggio et al. 1989; Schein et al. 1989). Because of the rarity of ulcerative keratitis, controlled prospective clinical studies would require a very large sample size to determine the effect of lens type on this response. To date, such a study has not been conducted to compare the incidence of these events with conventional- and disposable-lens extended wear. A number of retrospective case-control studies based on practitioner surveys or patient attendance at eye hospitals have been reported. Lack of the use of standard clinical definitions for sterile and infectious keratitis and the absence of positive cultures in many cases of presumed infectious keratitis create difficulty in making comparisons, however.

The normal open-eye defense mechanisms against infection include an intact corneal epithelium, blinking, tear film flushing, and antimicrobial components of the tear film. Some of these mechanisms are absent or impaired during eye closure. Also, there is increased microbial load on the conjunctiva and lid margins with eye closure, imparting stress on the ocular defenses and immune system (Ramachandran et al. 1995).

Undoubtedly, the major risk factor for corneal infection during hydrogel lens wear is overnight use of lenses (Weissman et al. 1984; Schein et al. 1989, 1994). The risk of ulcerative keratitis increases with each additional consecutive night of lens wear (Schein et al. 1989, 1994). The principal reason for this finding is believed to be the impaired resistance of the epithelium to microbial invasion induced by corneal hypoxia. Other factors include inoculation by contaminated solutions or the patient's fingers, improper lens disinfection, change to a warm climate, improper lens fit, lens manipulation during wear, ocular trauma, diabetes, upper respiratory tract infection or influenza, smoking, and poor patient instruction.

Cases of microbial, fungal, and amebic keratitis have been documented with both conventional- and disposable-lens extended wear. The risk of ulcerative keratitis with hydrogel lens extended wear is greater than that for rigid gas-permeable lens extended wear (Franks et al. 1988; Bates et al. 1989). If hypoxia is a major factor, one intuitively would predict a similar incidence with conventional and disposable lenses of similar oxygen transmissibility. The triggering mechanism is not hypoxia in all cases, however, because a case of infectious keratitis has been reported during silicone elastomer lens wear (Adams et al. 1983), and similar incidences are seen for polymethyl methacrylate and rigid gas-permeable lens daily wear (Poggio et al. 1989; Schein and Poggio 1990; Stapleton et al. 1993).

In 1992, two studies (Buehler et al. 1992; Matthews et al. 1992) showed an increased risk of corneal infection with disposable lenses. However, a reanalysis at one of these institutions (Schein et al. 1994) found no significant difference in the incidence of infectious keratitis between disposable- and conventional-lens extended wear, even though the average number of consecutive nights of lens wear was four times greater for the disposable-lens wearers studied. Recent studies of contact lens–induced keratitis in Sweden and the United Kingdom also have shown no difference in risk between disposable- and conventional-lens extended wear (Poggio and Abelson 1993; Nilsson and Montan 1994a, b).

Of the possible contributing factors, two sources of contamination—lens care products and the lens case—are removed from the system with disposable-lens extended wear. Disposable extended-wear lenses may also be associated with reduced lens spoilation. Other contributing factors are essentially similar for disposable- and conventional-lens extended wear. There have been reports of inadequate lens care regimens being recommended to disposable-lens wearers to enhance convenience, including the absence of surfactant cleaning and friction cleaning and use of an inadequate disinfection solution (McLaughlin et al. 1989; Efron et al. 1991). In such cases, infectious keratitis should not be attributed solely to the lens type.

The mechanisms that promote or inhibit bacterial adherence to the cornea during open- and closed-eye conditions are not well understood. In vitro assays are being conducted to identify agents that may be used to inhibit microbial adherence to the corneal epithelium, presumed to be the first step in corneal infection. The composition of bacterial biofilms secreted onto lens surfaces and the resistance they impart also are under investigation. Further work is required to determine the true relative risk of corneal infection for those who wear disposable and conventional lenses on an extended-wear basis.

COMPLICATION RATES

For purposes of comparison, investigators often group discontinuations due to adverse events, ocular structural changes, and discomfort to determine complication rates for various lens types and wear modes. Several investigators have reported lower overall complication rates with disposable and frequent-replacement lenses compared with conventional lenses for both daily and extended wear.

Ames and Cameron (1989) reported a significant reduction in both the signs and symptoms of redness, stinging, lens awareness, and itching during extended wear of lenses replaced every 3 months compared with lenses worn without planned replacement. Josephson et al. (1990) compared the extended-wear performance of disposable lenses on a weekly replacement schedule with a variety of conventional unreplaced lens types on a weekly disinfection schedule in fellow eyes. The overall performance in terms of ocular physiology was not significantly different after 1 and 6 weeks of lens wear, although there was a subjective preference for the regularly replaced lens.

Roth (1990) compared the extended-wear complication rates for disposable lenses replaced every 2 weeks and conventional unreplaced thin and ultrathin lenses. The complication rate was lower for disposable lenses, at 8% versus 20%. Marshall et al. (1992) also reported a lower complication rate for disposable-lens extended wear compared with conventional-lens extended wear. They noted a greater frequency of symptoms and signs related to lens deposits during conventional-lens extended wear.

Poggio and Abelson (1993) also found that the prevalence of complications with disposable-lens extended wear was significantly lower than that for conventional-lens extended wear but not significantly different from that of conventional-lens daily wear. Disposable-lens extended wear was associated with significantly fewer reports of symptoms, fewer unscheduled visits, and a longer wearing time compared with both conventional-lens daily and extended wear. In addition, in a large-scale study of complication rates in Japanese contact lens wearers, Hamano et al. (1994) found that the overall rate of corneal complications with disposable lenses worn on an extended-wear schedule (by 92.5% of the wearers) was lower than that for daily wear of conventional lenses.

In a retrospective analysis of subjective and objective complications with conventional-lens and disposable-lens extended wear, Boswall et al. (1993) found a lower complication rate with disposable-lens wear, although the average wearing time before overnight lens removal also was significantly lower than that for conventional-lens wear. Another noteworthy finding of this investigation was the significantly higher number of patients with a history of contact lens–related complications in the group fitted for disposable-lens extended wear, compared with the group fitted for conventional-lens extended wear. This trend also may occur in other retrospective or prospective studies and should be taken into account when complication rates are compared because there is evidence for some degree of patient sensitization with respect to inflammatory ocular events, regardless of lens type or wear schedule.

A MODEL FOR SAFE HYDROGEL LENS EXTENDED WEAR

Hypoxia, inflammation, and infection will continue to occur with current hydrogel lens extended wear, regardless of lens replacement schedules. Researchers at our institution have generated a model for achieving safe, continuous hydrogel lens wear based on the interaction of these three factors. The model predicts that all three elements are interrelated to a certain degree.

According to this model, the development of soft lenses with high oxygen permeability will reduce hypoxic complications significantly, although these complications will not be eliminated completely. Similarly, the incidence of inflammation and infection will be reduced, although to a lesser extent. Anti-inflammatory and anti-infective strategies must be researched and developed concurrently to achieve safe, comfortable, continuous wear of soft contact lenses.

CONCLUSION

The introduction of disposable lenses led to a resurgence in the popularity of extended wear. Hypoxic, inflammatory, and infectious complications soon were documented with this new modality, however, dispelling the belief that these lenses are the ultimate solution for safe, continuous wear. At the same time, clinical experience also suggested an improvement over conventional-lens extended wear in some areas, particularly in tissue responses to lens deposition and patient satisfaction.

Hypoxia underlies most of the complications associated with hydrogel lens extended wear, and regular lens replacement of conventional or disposable lenses has no effect on this problem. All current hydrogel lenses create hypoxic stress, resulting in significant morphologic and functional corneal compromise. Conventional and disposable-lens extended wear induces hypoxic changes to a similar extent, including increased anaerobic metabolism, stromal acidosis, overnight corneal swelling, residual daytime corneal edema, microcysts, vacuoles, striae, folds, blebs, and polymegathism. Some controversy remains as to the relative incidence of corneal staining, neovascularization, infiltrates, and sterile and infectious keratitis for disposable- and conventional-lens extended wear. However, disposable-lens extended wear induces significantly fewer contact lens–induced acute red eye reactions, compared with conventional-lens extended wear.

It is possible that some complications associated with disposable-lens use could be reduced further with an increased lens-parameter range, permitting greater lens movement for some patients. Lens movement is essential for the removal of the products of corneal metabolism, tear film debris, exfoliated epithelial cells, and inflammatory mediators. The recommended fitting philosophy for hydrogel lens extended wear is to achieve maximum sustained lens movement while maintaining comfort and stable vision.

Our recommendations for care and maintenance of conventional hydrogel lenses for extended wear include replacement every month or every 3 months, surfactant cleaning, use of unpreserved saline and a proven disinfectant, and regular enzymatic cleaning. Instillation of an in-eye lubricant (unit dose) before and after overnight lens wear also is advised. For disposable-lens extended wear, we recommend weekly lens replacement and the use of in-eye lubricant morning and night. Flexible or intermittent overnight wear is a safer alternative to extended or continuous wear. Flexible overnight wear allows the cornea to return regularly to a more normal thickness and decreases the contact time between the post-lens tear debris and contaminated lenses and the cornea, thereby decreasing the risk of inflammation or infection. The lens cleaning and disinfection routine recommended for conventional-lens extended wear also applies during disposable-lens flexible extended wear and is an essential step before lens reinsertion.

Very thin, high-water-content hydrogel lenses provide improved oxygen transmissibility but not to the level required to maintain normal epithelial aerobic metabolism. In addition, these lenses can induce corneal desiccation, have inadequate durability, and are difficult to handle. Silicone elastomer lenses have yet to attain successful clinical performance in terms of surface chemistry, comfort, and maintenance of lens movement for any group of patients except aphakic infants and children. Other nonhydrogel materials with high oxygen permeability are currently being tested in short- and long-term clinical trials and are showing some promise. It must also be remembered that corneal compromise is not only a function of impaired oxygen supply but is likely also to be affected by carbon dioxide accumulation in the tissue. Hence, adequate carbon dioxide transmissibility is another requirement for a successful lens polymer.

Although clinical research findings and in vitro investigations have allowed the development of one model for safe extended wear, we do not have the complete picture yet. The model implies that maximizing lens oxygen transmissibility will not eradicate inflammatory and infectious events during overnight wear. The triggering mechanisms for these reactions have to be identified, but it is likely that the closed-eye environment holds the key to understanding these stimuli. Ongoing research in this area and investigations to identify the activators and inhibitors of corneal inflammation may allow the development of pharmaceutical agents that could be incorporated into a lens material or lens care system. This research also could allow the development of predictive tests whereby patients at risk are detected before they attempt extended wear.

Extended wear of current hydrogel polymers causes subtle long-term tissue changes that have serious implications. Overall, the risk-to-benefit ratio is reduced for disposable-lens extended wear in comparison with conventional-lens extended wear. Although not discussed within the confines of this chapter, the safest currently available option for extended wear is undoubtedly the high-Dk, rigid gas-permeable lens. New "soft" materials with high oxygen transmissibilities, anti-inflammatory and anti-infective components, and improved wettability ultimately are required to provide both safety and comfort during extended wear.

REFERENCES

Adams CP, Cohen EJ, Laibson PR, et al. Corneal ulcers in patients with cosmetic extended-wear contact lenses. Am J Ophthalmol 1983;96:705.

Alio JL, Ayala MJ, Muler E, et al. Treatment of experimental acute corneal inflammation with inhibitors of the oxidative metabolism. Ophthalmic Res 1993;25:331.

Allansmith MR, Korb DR, Greiner JV, et al. Giant papillary conjunctivitis in contact lens wearers. Am J Ophthalmol 1977;83:697.

Ames KS, Cameron MH. The efficacy of regular lens replacement in extended wear. Int Contact Lens Clin 1989;16:104.

Ang JHB, Efron N. Carbon dioxide permeability of contact lens materials. Int Contact Lens Clin 1989;16:48.

Aswad MJ, John T, Barza M, et al. Bacterial adherence to extended wear soft contact lenses. Ophthalmology 1990;97:296.

Bachman WG, Wilson G. Essential ions for maintenance of the corneal epithelial surface. Invest Ophthalmol Vis Sci 1985;26:1484.

Baleriola-Lucas C, Grant T, Newton-Howes J, et al. Enumeration and identification of bacteria on hydrogel lenses from asymptomatic patients and those experiencing adverse reactions with extended wear. Invest Ophthalmol Vis Sci 1991;32(suppl):739.

Ballow M, Donshik PC, Rapaz P, Samartino L. Tear lactoferrin levels in patients with external inflammatory ocular disease. Invest Ophthalmol Vis Sci 1987;28:543.

Barr JT. Contact lenses and vision. The annual report. Contact Lens Spectrum 1997;12:21.

Barr JT, Lapple WJ, Snyder AC, et al. Evaluation of contact lenses by microbial enumeration and protein determination. Am J Optom Physiol Opt 1988;65:476.

Basu PK, Minta JO. Chemotactic migration of leukocytes through corneal layers: an in vitro study. Can J Ophthalmol 1976;11:235.

Bates AK, Morris RJ, Stapleton F, et al. "Sterile" corneal infiltrates in contact lens wearers. Eye 1989;3:803.

Baum J. A relatively dry eye during sleep. Cornea 1990;9:1.

Baum J, Barza M. *Pseudomonas* keratitis and extended wear soft contact lenses. Arch Ophthalmol 1990;108:663.

Bazan NG, Bazan HEP. Ocular Responses to Inflammation and the Triggering of Wound Healing: Lipid Mediators, Proto-Oncogenes, Gene Expression, and Neuromodulation. In NG Bazan (ed), Lipid Mediators in Eye Inflammation. New Trends in Lipid Mediators Research. Basel: Karger, 1990;168.

Bergmanson JPG. Histopathological analysis of the corneal epithelium after contact lens wear. J Am Optom Assoc 1987;58:812.

Bergmanson JPG. Histopathological examination of corneas with contact lens-induced endothelial polymegethism. Invest Ophthalmol Vis Sci 1990;31(suppl):549.

Bergmanson JPG. Histopathological analysis of corneal endothelial polymegethism. Cornea 1992;11:133.

Bergmanson JPG, Chu LW-F. Corneal response to rigid contact lens wear. Br J Ophthalmol 1982;66:667.

Bergmanson JPG, Ruben CM, Chu LW-F. Epithelial morphological response to soft hydrogel contact lenses. Br J Ophthalmol 1985;69:373.

Bergstresser PR, Fletcher CR, Streilein JW. Surface densities of Langerhans cells in relation to rodent epidermal sites with special immunologic properties. J Invest Dermatol 1980;74:77.

Berman M, Winthrop S, Ausprunk D, et al. Plasminogen activator (urokinase) causes vascularization of the cornea. Invest Ophthalmol Vis Sci 1982;22:191.

Bonanno JA, Polse KA. Central and peripheral corneal swelling accompanying soft lens extended wear. Am J Optom Physiol Opt 1985;62:74.

Bonanno JA, Polse KA. Corneal acidosis during contact lens wear: effects of hypoxia and CO_2. Invest Ophthalmol Vis Sci 1987a;28:1514.

Bonanno JA, Polse KA. Measurement of in vivo human corneal stromal pH: open and closed eye. Invest Ophthalmol Vis Sci 1987b;28:522.

Boswall GJ, Ehlers WH, Luistro A, et al. A comparison of conventional and disposable extended wear contact lenses. CLAO J 1993;19:158.

Bourassa S, Benjamin WJ. Transient corneal surface "microdeposits" and associated epithelial surface pits occurring with gel contact lens extended wear (a case report). Int Contact Lens Clin 1988;15:338.

Bucci FA, Lopatynsky MO, Jenkins PL, et al. Comparison of the clinical performance of the ACU-VUE® disposable contact lens and CSI lens in patients with giant papillary conjunctivitis. Am J Ophthalmol 1993;115:454.

Buehler PO, Schein OD, Stamler JF, et al. The increased risk of ulcerative keratitis among disposable soft contact lens users. Arch Ophthalmol 1992;110:1555.

Butrus SI, Klotz SA, Misra RP. The adherence of *Pseudomonas aeruginosa* to soft contact lenses. Ophthalmology 1987;94:1310.

Carney LG, Brennan NA. Time course of corneal oxygen uptake during contact lens wear. CLAO J 1988;14:151.

Carney LG, Hill RM. Human tear pH. Arch Ophthalmol 1976;94:821.

Carubelli R, Nodkuist R, Remsey J. Role of active oxygen species in corneal ulceration. Cornea 1990;2:161.

Cassel G, Groden LR. New thoughts on ocular neovascularization: a neurally controlled regenerative process? Ann Ophthalmol 1984;16:138.

Catania LJ. Sterile infiltrates vs. infectious keratitis: worlds apart. Int Contact Lens Clin 1987;14:412.

Chandler JW, Leder R, Kaufman HE, Caldwell JR. Quantitative determinations of complement components and immunoglobulins in tears and aqueous humor. Invest Ophthalmol Vis Sci 1974;13:151.

Cheng KH, Kok JHC, von Mil C, Kijlstra A. Selective binding of a 30-kilodalton protein to disposable hydrophilic contact lenses. Invest Ophthalmol Vis Sci 1990;31:2244.

Chignell AH, Easty DL, Chesterton JR, Thomsitt J. Marginal ulceration of the cornea. Br J Ophthalmol 1970;54:433.

Chiou GCY, Chang MS. Ocular Inflammation Induced by Lens Protein and Its Prevention with New Agents. In NG Bazan (ed), Lipid Mediators in Eye Inflammation. New Trends in Lipid Mediators Research. Basel: Karger, 1990;94.

Cogan DG. Vascularization of the cornea. Arch Ophthalmol 1949;41:406.

Connor CG, Zagrod ME. Contact lens-induced corneal endothelial polymegathism: functional significance and possible mechanisms. Am J Optom Physiol Opt 1986;63:539.

Crook T. Corneal infiltrates with red eye related to duration of extended wear. J Am Optom Assoc 1985;56:698.

Cutter GR, Chalmers RL, Roseman M. The clinical presentation, prevalence, and risk factors of focal corneal infiltrates in soft contact lens wearers. CLAO J 1996;22:30.

Dart JKG. Complications of extended wear hydrogel contact lenses. Contax 1986;March/April:11.

Dart JKG, Badenoch PR. Bacterial adherence to contact lenses. CLAO J 1986;12:220.

Davson H. The Physiology of the Eye (3rd ed). London: Churchill Livingstone, 1972;68.

DiGaetano M, Stern GA, Zam ZS. The pathogenesis of contact lens–associated *Pseudomonas aeruginosa* corneal ulceration: II. An animal model. Cornea 1986;5:155.

Dohlman CH, Boruchoff A, Mobilia EF. Complications in the use of soft contact lenses in corneal disease. Arch Ophthalmol 1973;90:367.

Donshik P, Weinstock FJ, Wechsler S, et al. Disposable hydrogel contact lenses for extended wear. CLAO J 1988;14:191.

Duran JA, Refojo MF, Gipson IK, Kenyon KR. *Pseudomonas* attachment to new hydrogel contact lenses. Arch Ophthalmol 1987;105:106.

Dutt RM, Stocker EG, Wolff CH, et al. A morphologic and fluorophotometric analysis of the corneal endothelium in long-term extended wear soft contact lens wearers. CLAO J 1989;15:121.

Efron N. Clinical management of corneal edema. Contact Lens Spectrum 1986;1(12):13.

Efron N. Vascular response of the cornea to contact lens wear. J Am Optom Assoc 1987;58:836.

Efron N, Brennan NA, O'Brien KA, Murphy PJ. Surface dehydration of hydrogel contact lenses. Clin Exp Optom 1986;69:219.

Efron N, Veys J. Defects in disposable contact lenses can compromise ocular integrity. Int Contact Lens Clin 1992;19:8.

Efron N, Wohl A, Toma NG, et al. *Pseudomonas* corneal ulcers associated with daily wear of disposable hydrogel contact lenses. Int Contact Lens Clin 1991;18:46.

Elgebaly SA, Gillies C, Forouhar F, et al. An in-vitro model of leukocyte mediated injury to the corneal epithelium. Curr Eye Res 1985;4:31.

Eliason JA. Leucocytes and experimental corneal vascularization. Invest Ophthalmol Vis Sci 1978;17:1087.

Ellingsworth LP, Nakayama D, Segravini P, et al. Transforming growth factor-betas are equipotent growth inhibitors of interleukin-1 induced thymocyte proliferation. Cell Immunol 1988;114:41.

Epstein AB, Donnenfeld ED. Epithelial microcysts associated with the ACUVUE® disposable CL. Contact Lens Forum 1989;14:35.

Farris RL, Kubota Z, Mishima S. Epithelial decompensation with corneal contact lens wear. Arch Ophthalmol 1971;85:651.

Farris RL, Takahashi GH, Donn A. Oxygen flux across the in vivo rabbit cornea. Arch Ophthalmol 1965;74:679.

Fleiszig SMJ, Efron N, Pier GB. Extended contact lens wear enhances *Pseudomonas aeruginosa* adherence to human corneal epithelium. Invest Ophthalmol Vis Sci 1992;33:2908.

Fowler SA, Greiner JV, Allansmith MR. Attachment of bacteria to soft contact lenses. Arch Ophthalmol 1979;97:659.

Franks WA, Adams GGW, Dart JKG, Minassian O. Relative risks of different types of contact lenses. Br Med J 1988;297:524.

Freeman RD. Oxygen consumption by the component layers of the cornea. J Physiol 1972;225:15.

Freeman RD, Fatt I. Environmental influences on ocular temperature. Invest Ophthalmol Vis Sci 1973;12:596.

Fromer CH, Klintworth GK. An evaluation of the role of leukocytes in the pathogenesis of experimentally induced corneal vascularization: III. Studies related to the vasoproliferative capability of polymorphonuclear leucocytes and lymphocytes. Am J Pathol 1976;82:157.

Gauthier C, Holden B, Terry R. Can contact lens wearers be correctly identified from their "appearance?" Invest Ophthalmol Vis Sci 1992;33(suppl):1294.

Gilbard JP, Cohen GR, Gray KL, et al. The effect of eye closure with sleep on the human tear film. Invest Ophthalmol Vis Sci 1988;29(suppl):47.

Gordon A, Kracher GP. Corneal infiltrates and extended wear contact lenses. J Am Optom Assoc 1985;56:198.

Grant T. Clinical Aspects of Planned Replacement and Disposable Lenses. In C Kerr (ed), The Contact Lens Year Book. Hythe, UK: Medical and Scientific Publishing, 1991;15.

Grant T, Chong MS, Holden BA. Which is best for the eye: daily wear, 2 nights or 6 nights? Am J Optom Physiol Opt 1988a;65(suppl):40P.

Grant T, Kotow M, Holden BA. Hydrogel extended wear: current performance and future options. Contax 1987;May:5.

Grant T, Chong MS, Holden BA. Management of GPC with daily disposable lenses. Am J Optom Physiol Opt 1988b;65(suppl):94P.

Grant T, Holden BA, Rechberger J, Chong MS. Contact lens-related papillary conjunctivitis (CLPC): influence of protein accumulation and replacement frequency. Invest Ophthalmol Vis Sci 1989;30(suppl):166.

Grant T, Terry R, Holden BA. Extended Wear of Hydrogel Lenses: Clinical Problems and Their Management. In M Harris (ed), Problems in Optometry, Vol 2, No 4. Philadelphia: Lippincott, 1990;599.

Gruber E. The disposable contact lens: a new concept in extended wear. CLAO J 1988;14:195.

Hamano H, Hori M, Hirayama K, et al. Influence of soft and hard contact lenses on the cornea. Aust J Optom 1975;58:326.

Hamano H, Hori M, Hamano T, et al. Effects of contact lens wear on mitosis of corneal epithelium and lactate content of aqueous humor of rabbit. Jpn J Ophthalmol 1983;27:451.

Hamano H, Hori M, Hirayama K, Mitsunaga S. Fundamental information of contact lens wear on the eye. J Jpn Contact Lens Soc 1976;18:1.

Hamano H, Watanabe K, Hamano T, et al. A study of the complications induced by conventional and disposable contact lenses. CLAO J 1994;20:103.

Harris JK, Shovlin JP, Pascicci SE, et al. Keratitis associated with extended wear of disposable contact lenses. Contact Lens Spectrum 1989;4(4):55.

Hart GW. Corneal Proteoglycans. In DS McDevitt (ed), Cell Biology of the Eye. New York: Academic, 1982;1.

Hart DE, DePaolis M, Ratner BD, Mateo NB. Surface analysis of hydrogel contact lenses by ESCA. CLAO J 1993;19:169.

Henriquez AS. New information on giant papillary conjunctivitis and corneal infiltrates. Contact Lens J 1987;15:10.

Herman JP. Clinical management of GPC. Contact Lens Spectrum 1987;2(11):24.

Hill RM. Oxygen uptake of the cornea following contact lens removal. J Am Optom Assoc 1965;36:913.

Hill RM. How the cornea "takes the heat." Int Contact Lens Clin 1978;5:65.

Hodd NFB. An analysis of permanent wear success. Optician 1977;174(4491):23.

Hogan MJ, Zimmerman LE. The Cornea and Sclera. In MJ Hogan, LE Zimmerman (eds), Ophthalmic Pathology—An Atlas and Textbook. Philadelphia: Saunders, 1962;277.

Holden BA. Corneal requirements for extended wear: an update. CLAO J 1988;14:220.

Holden BA. The Glenn A. Fry award lecture 1988: the ocular response to contact lens wear. Optom Vis Sci 1989;66:717.

Holden BA, Kotow M, Swarbrick HA. The current status of extended wear. Contax 1986c;March/April:21.

Holden BA, La Hood D, Grant T, et al. Gram-negative bacteria can induce contact lens–induced acute red eye (CLARE) responses. CLAO J 1996;22:47.

Holden BA, McNally JJ, Mertz GW, Swarbrick HA. Topographical corneal oedema. Acta Ophthalmol (Copenh) 1985e;63:684.

Holden BA, Mertz GW. Critical oxygen levels to avoid corneal edema for daily and extended wear contact lenses. Invest Ophthalmol Vis Sci 1984;25:1161.

Holden BA, Mertz GW, McNally JJ. Corneal swelling response to contact lenses worn under extended wear conditions. Invest Ophthalmol Vis Sci 1983;24:218.

Holden BA, Polse KA, Fonn D, Mertz GW. Effects of cataract surgery on corneal function. Invest Ophthalmol Vis Sci 1982;22:343.

Holden BA, Ross R, Jenkins J. Hydrogel contact lenses impede carbon dioxide efflux from the human cornea. Curr Eye Res 1987;6:1283.

Holden BA, Sweeney DF. The oxygen tension and temperature of the superior palpebral conjunctiva. Acta Ophthalmol (Copenh) 1985;63:100.

Holden BA, Sweeney DF. The significance of the microcyst response: a review. Optom Vis Sci 1991;68:703.

Holden BA, Sweeney D, Jenkins J, et al. Factors contributing to contact lens induced edema. Am J Optom Physiol Opt 1981;58(suppl):1010.

Holden BA, Sweeney DF, Sanderson G. The minimum precorneal oxygen tension to avoid corneal edema. Invest Ophthalmol Vis Sci 1984;25:476.

Holden BA, Sweeney DF, Seger R. Epithelial erosions caused by thin high water content lenses. Clin Exp Optom 1986a;69:103.

Holden BA, Sweeney DF, Swarbrick HA, et al. The vascular response to long-term extended contact lens wear. Clin Exp Optom 1986b;69:112.

Holden BA, Sweeney DF, Vannas A, et al. Contact lens induced endothelial polymegethism. Invest Ophthalmol Vis Sci 1985d;26(suppl):275.

Holden BA, Sweeney DF, Vannas A, et al. Effects of long-term extended contact lens wear on the human cornea. Invest Ophthalmol Vis Sci 1985a;26:1489.

Holden BA, Vannas A, Nilsson K, et al. Epithelial and endothelial effects from the extended wear of contact lenses. Curr Eye Res 1985b;4:739.

Holden BA, Williams L, Zantos SG. The etiology of transient endothelial changes in the human cornea. Invest Ophthalmol Vis Sci 1985c;26:1354.

Huff J. Contact lens–induced edema in vitro. Invest Ophthalmol Vis Sci 1990;31:1288.

Humphreys JA, Larke JR. Micro-epithelial cysts and extended contact lens wear. J Br Contact Lens Assoc 1980;3:138.

Huth SW, Lannom CS, Lannom S. Effect of in vivo and in vitro surface protein deposits on the oxygen permeability of polyhydroxyethylmethacrylate gel contact lenses. Am J Optom Physiol Optics 1984;61:232.

Huth SW, Miller MJ, Leopold IH. Calcium and protein in tears: diurnal variation. Arch Ophthalmol 1981;99:1628.

Imre G. Neovascularization of the Eye. In JH Bellows (ed), Contemporary Ophthalmology. Baltimore: Williams & Wilkins, 1972;88.

Ivins PG. Early impressions of a disposable system. Optician 1988;195(5147):27.

Jackson WB, Gilmore NJ. Ocular immunology: a review (second of two parts). Can J Ophthalmol 1981;16:59.

Jager MJ, Atherron A, Bradley D, Streilein JW. Herpetic stromal keratitis in mice: less reversibility in the presence of Langerhans cells in the central cornea. Curr Eye Res 1990;10:69.

Jensen JA, Hunt TK, Scheuenstuhl H, Banda MJ. Effect of lactate, pyruvate, and pH on secretion of angiogenesis and mitogenesis factors by macrophages. Lab Invest 1986;54:574.

Josephson JE, Caffery BE. Infiltrative keratitis in hydrogel lens wearers. Int Contact Lens Clin 1979;6:223.

Josephson JE, Zantos S, Caffery B, Herman JP. Differentiation of corneal complications observed in contact lens wearers. J Am Optom Assoc 1988;59:679.

Josephson JA, Caffery BE. Proposed hypothesis for corneal infiltrates, microabrasions, and red eye associated with extended wear. Optom Vis Sci 1989;66:192.

Josephson JE, Caffery BE, Campbell I, Slomovic AR. Disposable contact lenses vs. contact lens maintenance for extended wear. CLAO J 1990;16:184.

Kamiya C, Mikami M, Iwata S. Biochemical studies on lactic acid formation in the rabbit cornea during oxygen-permeable hard contact lens wear. J Jpn Contact Lens Soc 1982;24:253.

Kanai A, Kaufman H. Electron microscopic studies of swollen corneal stroma. Ann Ophthalmol 1973;5:178.

Kangas TA, Edelhauser HF, Twining SS, O'Brien WJ. Loss of stromal glycosaminoglycans during corneal edema. Invest Ophthalmol Vis Sci 1990;31:1994.

Kaye GI, Edelhauser HF, Stern ME, et al. Further Studies of the Effect of Perfusion with a Calcium-Free Medium on the Rabbit Cornea: Extraction of Stromal Components. In JG Hollyfield (ed), The Structure of the Eye. Amsterdam: Elsevier, 1982;271.

Kehrl JH, Wakefield LM, Roberts AB, et al. Production of transforming growth factor beta by human T lymphocytes and its potential role in regulation of T cell growth. J Exp Med 1986;163:1037.

Kenyon E, Polse KA, Seger RG. Influence of wearing schedule on extended-wear complications. Ophthalmology 1986;93:231.

Kenyon E, Polse KA, Mandell RB. Rigid contact lens adherence: incidence, severity and recovery. J Am Optom Assoc 1988;59:168.

Klareskog L, Forsum U, Tjernlund UM, et al. Expression of Ia antigen-like molecules on cells in the corneal epithelium. Invest Ophthalmol Vis Sci 1979;3:310.

Klintworth GK, Burger PC. Neovascularization of the cornea: current concepts of its pathogenesis. Int Ophthalmol Clin 1983;23:27.

Klyce SD, Bernegger O. Epithelial hypoxia, lactate production and stromal oedema. Invest Ophthalmol Vis Sci 1978;17(suppl):227.

Knighton DR, Hunt TK, Scheuenstuhl H, et al. Oxygen tension regulates the expression of angiogenesis factor by macrophages. Science 1983;221:1283.

Koetting RA, Metz CJ, Seibel DB. Clinical impressions of extended wear success relative to patient age. J Am Optom Assoc 1988;59:164.

Kotow M, Grant T, Holden BA. Avoiding ocular complications during hydrogel extended wear. Int Contact Lens Clin 1987b;14:95.

Kotow M, Holden BA, Grant T. The value of regular replacement of low water content contact lenses for extended wear. J Am Optom Assoc 1987a;58:461.

Kwok LS. Review: the effect of contact lens wear on the electrophysiology of the corneal epithelium. Aust J Optom 1983;66:138.

La Hood D, Sweeney DF, Holden BA. Overnight corneal edema with hydrogel, rigid gas-permeable and silicone elastomer contact lenses. Int Contact Lens Clin 1988;15:149.

Leahy CD, Mandell RB, Lin ST. Initial in vivo tear protein deposition on individual hydrogel contact lenses. Optom Vis Sci 1990;67:504.

Leibowitz HM. Inflammation of the Cornea: Basic Principles. In HM Leibowitz (ed), Corneal Disorders: Clinical Diagnosis and Management. Philadelphia: Saunders, 1984;265.

Lemp MA, Gold JB. The effects of extended-wear hydrophilic contact lenses on the human corneal epithelium. Am J Ophthalmol 1986;101:274.

Lin S, Mandell B. Corneal blotting from extended wear. Contact Lens Spectrum 1991;6(2):25.

Lin ST, Mandell RB, Leahy CD, Newell JO. Protein accumulation on disposable extended wear lenses. CLAO J 1991;17:44.

MacRae SM, Matsuda M, Shellans S. Corneal endothelial changes associated with contact lens wear. CLAO J 1989;15:82.

MacRae SM, Andre M, Matsuda M, Phillips D. Comparison of daily wear (DW) vs. extended wear (EW) soft endothelial morphology in paired eyes. Invest Ophthalmol Vis Sci 1990;31(suppl):407.

MacRae SM, Matsuda M, Phillips DS. The long-term effects of polymethylmethacrylate contact lens wear on the corneal endothelium. Ophthalmology 1994;101:365.

MacRae SM, Matsuda M, Shellans S, Rich LF. The effects of hard and soft contact lenses on the corneal endothelium. Am J Ophthalmol 1986;102:50.

Madigan MC. Cat and monkey as models for extended hydrogel contact lens wear in humans. PhD thesis, University of New South Wales, Sydney, Australia, 1989.

Madigan MC, Holden BA. Reduced epithelial adhesion after extended contact lens wear correlates with reduced hemidesmosome density in cat cornea. Invest Ophthalmol Vis Sci 1992;33:314.

Madigan MC, Holden BA, Kwok LS. Extended wear of hydrogel contact lenses can compromise corneal epithelial adhesion. Curr Eye Res 1987;6:1257.

Madigan MC, Penfold PL, Holden BA, Billson FA. Ultrastructural features of contact lens–induced deep corneal neovascularization and associated stromal leucocytes. Cornea 1990;9:144.

Maguen E, Rosner I, Caroline P, et al. A retrospective study of disposable extended wear lenses in 100 patients: year 2. CLAO J 1992;18:229.

Maguen E, Rosner IR, Caroline P, et al. A retrospective study of disposable extended wear lenses in 100 patients: year 3. CLAO J 1994;20:179.

Maguen E, Tsai JC, Martinez M, et al. A retrospective study of disposable extended-wear lenses in 100 patients. Ophthalmology 1991;98:1685.

Mandell RB. Corneal edema and curvature changes from gel lenses. Int Contact Lens Clin 1975;2:88.

Mandell RB, Fatt I. Thinning of the human cornea on awakening. Nature 1965;208:292.

Marshall EC, Begley CG, Nguyen CHD. Frequency of complications among wearers of disposable and conventional soft contact lenses. Int Contact Lens Clin 1992;19:55.

Marshall J, Grindall J. Fine structure of the cornea and its development. Br J Ophthalmol 1978;98:320.

Matthews TD, Frazer DG, Minassian DC, et al. Risks of keratitis and patterns of use with disposable contact lenses. Arch Ophthalmol 1992;110:1559.

Maurice DM, Zauberman H, Michaelson IC. The stimulus to neovascularization in the cornea. Exp Eye Res 1966;5:168.

McLaughlin R, Kelly CG, Mauger TF. Corneal ulceration associated with disposable EW lenses. Contact Lens Spectrum 1989;4(3):57.

McLeish W, Rubsamen P, Atherton SS, Streilein JW. Immunobiology of Langerhans cells on the ocular surface: II. Role of central corneal Langerhans cells in stromal keratitis following experimental HSV-1 infection in mice. Reg Immunol 1989;2:236.

Mertz GW, Holden BA. Clinical implications of extended wear research. Can J Optom 1981;4:203.

Michielsen B, Kempeneers A, Houttequiet I, Missotten L. Disposable soft contact lenses. Contactologia 1990;12E:178.

Mikami M, Nakazawa M, Anan N, Iwata S. Studies on reaction of the anterior segment to the wearing of the contact lens: I. Lactate formation in the rabbit aqueous humor. J Jpn Contact Lens Soc 1981;23:186.

Millodot M. Effect of soft lenses on corneal sensitivity. Acta Ophthalmol (Copenh) 1974;52:603.

Millodot M, O'Leary DJ. Effect of oxygen deprivation on corneal sensitivity. Acta Ophthalmol (Copenh) 1980;58:434.

Millodot M, O'Leary DJ. Corneal fragility and its relationship to sensitivity. Acta Ophthalmol (Copenh) 1981;59:820.

Mishima S, Kaye GI, Takahashi GH, et al. The Function of the Corneal Endothelium in the Regulation of Corneal Hydration. In ME Langham (ed), The Cornea: Macromolecular Organization of a Connective Tissue. Baltimore: Johns Hopkins University Press, 1969;207.

Mizutani Y, Matsutaka H, Takemoto N, Mizutani Y. The effect of anoxia on the human cornea. Nippon Ganka Gakkai Zasshi 1983;87:644.

Molinari JF. Review: giant papillary conjunctivitis. Aust J Optom 1983;66:59.

Mondino BJ, Brown SI, Rabin BS, Bruno J. Alternate pathway activation of complement in a Proteus mirabilis ulceration of the cornea. Arch Ophthalmol 1978;96:1659.

Mondino BJ, Kowalski R, Ratajczak HV, et al. Rabbit model of phlyctenulosis and catarrhal infiltrates. Arch Ophthalmol 1981;99:891.

Mondino BJ, Rabin BS, Kessler E, et al. Corneal rings with gram-negative bacteria. Arch Ophthalmol 1977;95:2222.

Mondino BJ, Ratajczak HV, Goldberg DB, et al. Alternate and classical pathway components of complement in the normal cornea. Arch Ophthalmol 1980;98:346.

Newton-Howes JC, Durany N, Grant T, Holden BA. The distribution of proteins on the surface and in the matrix of hydrogel contact lenses. Optom Vis Sci 1989;66(suppl):90.

Nilsson SEG, Lindh H. Disposable contact lenses—a prospective study of clinical performance in flexible and extended wear. Contactologia 1990;12(2):80.

Nilsson SEG, Montan PG. The hospitalized cases of contact lens– induced keratitis in Sweden and their relation to lens type and wear schedule: results of a three-year retrospective study. CLAO J 1994a;20:97.

Nilsson SEG, Montan PG. The annualized incidence of contact lens induced keratitis in Sweden and its relation to lens type and wear schedule: results of a 3-month prospective study. CLAO J 1994b;20:225.

O'Leary DJ, Millodot M. Abnormal epithelial fragility in diabetes and contact lens wear. Acta Ophthalmol (Copenh) 1981;59:827.

O'Leary DJ, Wilson G, Bergmanson J. The influence of calcium in the tear-side perfusate on desquamation from the rabbit corneal epithelium. Curr Eye Res 1985;4:729.

O'Leary DJ, Wilson G, Henson DB. The effect of anoxia on the human corneal epithelium. Am J Optom Physiol Opt 1981;58:472.

O'Neal MR, Polse KA. Decreased endothelial pump function with aging. Invest Ophthalmol Vis Sci 1986;27:457.

O'Neal MR, Polse KA, Sarver MD. Corneal response to rigid and hydrogel lenses during eye closure. Invest Ophthalmol Vis Sci 1984;25:837.

Orsborn GN, Zantos SG. Corneal desiccation staining with thin high water content contact lenses. CLAO J 1988;14:81.

Pence NA. Corneal fatigue syndrome: the sequel. Contact Lens Spectrum 1988;3(12):64.

Phillips AJ. Extended-wear hydrogel lenses in the United Kingdom. Int Contact Lens Clin 1979;6:54.

Phillips AJ, Badenoch PR, Grutzmacher R, Roussel TJ. Microbial contamination of extended-wear contact lenses: an investigation of endotoxin as a cause of the acute ocular inflammation reaction. Int Eye Care 1986;2:469.

Poggio EC, Abelson M. Complications and symptoms in disposable extended wear lenses compared with conventional soft daily wear and soft extended wear lenses. CLAO J 1993;19:31.

Poggio EC, Glynn RJ, Schein OD, et al. The incidence of ulcerative keratitis among users of daily-wear and extended-wear soft contact lenses. N Engl J Med 1989;321:779.

Polse KA, Brand RJ, Cohen SR, Guillon M. Hypoxic effects on corneal morphology and function. Invest Ophthalmol Vis Sci 1990;31:1542.

Port M. A European multicentre extended wear study of the NewVues disposable contact lens. Contact Lens J 1991;19:86.

Prause JU, Brincker P, Dreyer V, Uangsted P. Light microscopical and scanning electron microscopical examinations of deposits on disposable constant wear lenses. Acta Ophthalmol (Copenh) 1988;66:3.

Ramachandran L, Sharma S, Sankaridurg PR, et al. Examination of the conjunctival microbiota after 8 hours of eye closure. CLAO J 1995;21:195.

Rao GN, Aquavella JV, Goldberg SH, Berk SL. Pseudophakic bullous keratopathy: relationship to preoperative corneal endothelial status. Ophthalmology 1984;91:1135.

Rapacz P, Tedesco J, Donshik PC, Ballow M. Tear lysozyme and lactoferrin levels in giant papillary conjunctivitis and vernal conjunctivitis. CLAO J 1988;14:207.

Refojo MF. Polymers, Dk, and contact lenses: now and in the future. CLAO J 1996;22:38.

Refojo MF, Leong F. Water-dissolved-oxygen permeability coefficients of hydrogel contact lenses and boundary layer effects. J Membr Sci 1979;4:415.

Rengstorff RH. Six-month soft lens replacements. Optom Manage 1983;19:43.

Reynolds RMP. Giant papillary conjunctivitis: a mechanical aetiology. Aust J Optom 1978;61:320.

Rietschel R, Wilson L. Ocular inflammation in patients using soft contact lenses. Arch Dermatol 1982;118:147.

Roth HW. Disposable lenses: indications and tolerance. Contactologia 1990;12E:173.

Sack RA, Jones B, Antignani A, et al. Specificity and biological activity of the protein deposited on the hydrogel surface. Invest Ophthalmol Vis Sci 1987;28:842.

Sack RA, Tan KO, Tan A. Diurnal tear cycle: evidence for a nocturnal inflammatory constitutive tear fluid. Invest Ophthalmol Vis Sci 1992;33:626.

Sack RA, Underwood PA, Tan KO, et al. Vitronectin: possible contribution to the closed-eye external host-defense mechanism. Ocular Immunol Inflamm 1993;1:327.

Samelsson B. Leukotrienes. A new group of biologically active compounds including SRS-A. Trends Pharmacol Sci 1980;9:227.

Sarver MD. Striate corneal lines among patients wearing hydrophilic contact lenses. Am J Optom 1971;48:762.

Schein OD, Buehler PO, Stamler JF, et al. The impact of overnight wear on the risk of contact lens–associated ulcerative keratitis. Arch Ophthalmol Vis Sci 1994;112:186.

Schein OD, Glynn RJ, Poggio EC, et al. The relative risk of ulcerative keratitis among users of daily-wear and extended-wear soft contact lenses. N Engl J Med 1989;321:773.

Schein OD, Poggio EC. Ulcerative keratitis in contact lens wearers. Cornea 1990;9(suppl 1):S55.

Schnider C, Zabkiewicz K, Holden BA. Unusual complications associated with rigid gas permeable extended wear. Int Contact Lens Clin 1988;15:124.

Schoessler JP, Barr J, Freson D. Corneal endothelial observations of silicone elastomer contact lens wearers. Int Contact Lens Clin 1984;11:337.

Schoessler JP, Orsborn GN. A theory of corneal endothelial polymegethism and aging. Curr Eye Res 1987;6:301.

Serdahl CL, Mannis MJ, Shapiro DR, et al. Infiltrative keratitis associated with disposable contact lenses. Am J Ophthalmol 1989;108:103.

Shams NBK, Huggins EM, Sigel MM. Interleukin-1 regulates the proliferation of leukocytes in human corneal cell-peripheral blood leukocyte cocultures. Cornea 1994;13:9.

Sholley MM, Gimbrone MA, Coltran RS. The effects of leucocyte depletion on corneal vascularization. Lab Invest 1978;38:32.

Shovlin JP. Sterile infiltrates associated with extended wear disposable contact lenses. Int Contact Lens Clin 1989;16:239.

Sibug ME, Datiles MB, Kashima K, et al. Specular microscopy studies on the corneal endothelium after cessation of contact lens wear. Cornea 1991;10:395.

Slusher MM, Myrvik QN, Lewis JC, Gristina AG. Extended wear lenses, biofilm, and bacterial adhesion. Arch Ophthalmol 1987;105:110.

Smolin G, Okumoto M, Nozik RA. The microbial flora in extended-wear soft contact-lens wearers. Am J Ophthalmol 1979;88:543.

Solomon OD. Corneal stress test for extended wear. CLAO J 1996;22:75.

Srinivasan BD, Jakobiec FA, Iwamoto T, De Voe G. Giant papillary conjunctivitis with ocular prostheses. Arch Ophthalmol 1979;97:892.

Stapleton F, Dart JKG, Minassian D. Risk factors with contact lens related suppurative keratitis. CLAO J 1993;19:204.

Stefansson E, Foulks GN, Hamilton RC. The effect of corneal contact lenses on the oxygen tension in the anterior chamber of the rabbit eye. Invest Ophthalmol Vis Sci 1987;28:1716.

Stern GA, Zam ZS. The pathogenesis of contact lens–associated *Pseudomonas aeruginosa* corneal ulceration: I. The effect of contact lens coatings on adherence of *Pseudomonas aeruginosa* to soft contact lenses. Cornea 1986;5:41.

Streilein JW, Toews GB, Bergstresser PR. Corneal allografts fail to express Ia antigens. Nature 1979;282:326.

Suchecki JK, Ehlers WH, Donshik PC. Peripheral corneal infiltrates associated with contact lens wear. CLAO J 1996;22:41.

Sweeney DF. Factors contributing to the human corneal oedema response. PhD thesis, School of Optometry, University of New South Wales, Sydney, Australia, 1991.

Sweeney DF. Corneal exhaustion syndrome with long-term wear of contact lenses. Optom Vis Sci 1992;69:601.

Sweeney DF, Grant T, Chong MS, et al. Recurrence of acute inflammatory conditions with hydrogel extended wear. Invest Ophthalmol Vis Sci 1993;34(suppl):1008.

Tan KO, Sack RA, Holden BA, Swarbrick HA. Temporal sequence of changes in tear film composition during sleep. Curr Eye Res 1993;12:1001.

Terry JE, Hill RM. Human tear osmotic pressure. Diurnal variation and the closed eye. Arch Ophthalmol 1978;96:139.

Tervo T, van Setten GB, Andersson R, et al. Contact lens wear is associated with the appearance of plasmin in the tear fluid—preliminary results. Graefes Arch Clin Exp Ophthalmol 1989;227:42.

Tervo T, van Setten GB, Joutsimo L, et al. Localization of proteolytic activity in contact lenses. Invest Ophthalmol Vis Sci 1990;31(suppl):406.

Tomlinson A, Haas DD. Changes in corneal thickness and circumcorneal vascularization with contact lens wear. Int Contact Lens Clin 1980;7:45.

Tsubota K, Hata S, Toda I, et al. Increase in corneal epithelial cell size with extended wear soft contact lenses depends on continuous wearing time. Br J Ophthalmol 1996;80:144.

Tsubota K, Yamada M. Corneal epithelial alterations induced by disposable contact lens wear. Ophthalmology 1992;99:1193.

Vajdic CM, Sweeney DF, Cornish R, et al. The incidence of idiopathic corneal infiltrates with disposable and rigid gas permeable daily and extended wear. Invest Ophthalmol Vis Sci 1995;36(suppl):S151.

van Klink F, Alizadeh H, He Y, et al. The role of contact lenses, trauma, and Langerhans cells in a Chinese hamster model of *Acanthamoeba* keratitis. Invest Ophthalmol Vis Sci 1993;34:1937.

van Setten GB, Tervo T, Andersson R, et al. Plasmin and epidermal growth factor in the tear fluid of contact-lens wearers: effect of wearing different types of contact lenses and association with clinical findings. Ophthalmic Res 1990;232:233.

Vannas A, Holden BA, Makitie J. The ultrastructure of contact lens–induced changes. Acta Ophthalmol (Copenh) 1984;62:320.

Vannas A, Makitie J, Sulonen J, et al. Contact lens–induced transient changes in corneal endothelium. Acta Ophthalmol (Copenh) 1981;59:552.

Vannas A, Sweeney DF, Holden BA, et al. Tear plasmin activity with contact lens wear. Curr Eye Res 1992;11:243.

Vansted P, Brincker P, Prause JU, Dreyer V. Short-term clinical trial of Danalens, a new disposable contact lens. Contactologia 1986;8:129.

Weissman BA, Mondino BJ, Pettit TH, Hofbauer JD. Corneal ulcers associated with extended-wear soft contact lenses. Am J Ophthalmol 1984;97:476.

Weissman BA, Schwartz SD, Lee DA. Oxygen transmissibility of disposable hydrogel contact lenses. CLAO J 1991;17:62.

Willcox MDP, Sweeney DF, Sharma S, et al. Culture negative peripheral ulcers are associated with bacterial contamination of contact lenses. Invest Ophthalmol Vis Sci 1995;36(suppl):S152.

Williams LJ. Transient endothelial changes in the in vivo human cornea. PhD thesis, University of New South Wales, Sydney, 1986.

Williams L, Holden BA. The bleb response of the endothelium decreases with extended wear of contact lenses. Clin Exp Optom 1986;69:90.

Wilson G, O'Leary DJ, Holden BA. Cell content of tears following overnight wear of a contact lens. Curr Eye Res 1989;8:329.

Woods CA. ACUVUE® in independent practice. Trans Br Contact Lens Assoc Conf 1989;6:33.

Yamaguchi H, Ogihara K, Kajita M, et al. Corneal endothelial cell changes in the early stage of contact lens wear. J Jpn Contact Lens Soc 1993;35:146.

Zantos SG. The ocular response to continuous wear of contact lenses. PhD thesis, School of Optometry, University of New South Wales, Sydney, 1981.

Zantos SG. Cystic formations in the corneal epithelium during extended wear of contact lenses. Int Contact Lens Clin 1983;10:128.

Zantos SG. Management of corneal infiltrates in extended wear contact lens patients. Int Contact Lens Clin 1984;11:604.

Zantos SG, Holden BA. Transient endothelial changes soon after wearing soft contact lenses. Am J Optom Physiol Opt 1977a;54:856.

Zantos SG, Holden BA. Research techniques and materials for continuous wear of contact lenses. Aust J Optom 1977b;60:86.

Zantos SG, Holden BA. Ocular changes associated with continuous wear of contact lenses. Aust J Optom 1978;61:418.

Zantos SG, Orsborn GN, Walter HC, Knoll HA. Studies on corneal staining with thin hydrogel contact lenses. J Br Contact Lens Assoc 1986;9:61.

7

Disposable Contact Lenses

Kiyoshi Watanabe and Hikaru Hamano

Many problems associated with contact lens wear, including allergic reactions and lens deposits, appear to be related to the length of the association between the eye and the lens. Other problems result from inadequate lens cleaning and contamination. Since 1990, in response to these shortcomings, the contact lens industry has developed a number of innovations, probably the most popular of which are the various types of disposable lenses. Although these lenses are worn for variable periods of time, they have in common the fact that they are replaced with new lenses at regular intervals, providing a "fresh start" for the patient and for the eye.

In this chapter, we discuss three types of disposable lenses and their patterns of wear in the United States and Japan. As used here, the term *disposable* refers to contact lenses that are discarded after a relatively short period of use (ranging from 1 day to approximately 12 weeks). The most common type, the *disposable extended-wear soft contact lens*, is worn continuously, day and night, for a period of up to 1 week, then is discarded. These lenses are not cleaned or disinfected and, once removed, are not replaced in the eye. A similar type of lens, removed periodically from the eye for cleaning and disinfection during the relatively short period of use (2–12 weeks), is termed the *frequent-replacement soft contact lens* (or planned-replacement soft contact lens). The newest entry into this field, the *daily-replacement disposable soft contact lens,* is worn for only 1 day, then is removed and discarded.

PATTERNS OF DISPOSABLE CONTACT LENS USE

United States

The first disposable extended-wear soft contact lens marketed in the United States was the ACUVUE lens, manufactured by Johnson & Johnson (Jacksonville, FL); this lens became available in 1987 and has enjoyed a rapidly expanding market share since that time. Later entries in this category are the SeeQuence lens from Bausch & Lomb (Rochester, NY), made by a spincasting procedure, and the NewVues lens from the CIBA Vision Corporation (Duluth, GA), made by a molding process. The

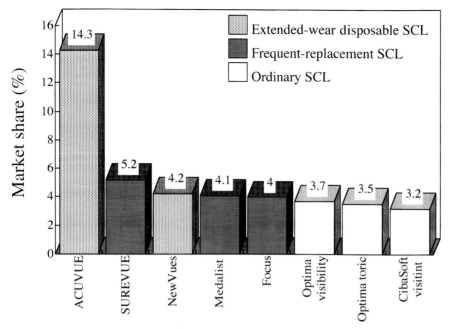

Figure 7.1 Market share of new fits for the eight most frequently prescribed soft contact lenses in the United States for the period October through December 1994. (SCL = soft contact lens.)

first frequent-replacement soft contact lens was the SUREVUE lens (also from Johnson & Johnson), which was designed to be disinfected chemically and discarded after 2 weeks of use; it was introduced in 1991. Daily-replacement disposable soft contact lenses, represented by the 1•DAY ACUVUE (Johnson & Johnson) and Occasions (Bausch & Lomb) lenses, first were marketed in 1994 at trial locations only on a limited basis.

During the period October through December 1994, the ACUVUE and NewVues extended-wear contact lenses made up approximately one-fifth of the new prescriptions for soft contact lenses in the United States (Figure 7.1). The major advantage of extended wear is that the wearer has good visual acuity from the moment he or she wakes up in the morning. Some patients dislike the sensation of dryness that accompanies the use of these lenses, however. In addition, the low oxygen permeability *(Dk)* of low-water-content disposable extended-wear soft contact lenses makes it impossible for some patients to wear them on a continuing basis.

Frequent-replacement disposable soft contact lenses, which were in second, fourth, and fifth places in terms of market share from October through December 1994, are expected to increase in popularity and eventually to replace many of the existing nondisposable types of soft contact lenses. Even now, low-water-content disposable extended-wear soft contact lenses often are used on a frequent-replacement basis for daily wear.

Daily-replacement disposable soft contact lenses still are new to the U.S. market, although the availability has been expanded greatly over the last year, and strong advertising and promotion efforts are under way to widen consumer interest. It is expected that the number of users of this lens will increase as supplies are assured and availability continues to expand.

Japan

As of 1993, there were approximately 10 million contact lens wearers in Japan, of whom 60–70% used hard lenses. To our knowledge, Japan is the only country in which hard lens wear is more common than is soft lens wear. In general, Japanese ophthalmologists believe hard contact lenses to be safer than soft contact lenses because of the low water content and poor oxygen permeability of the soft lenses. Although high-water-content soft contact lenses with improved Dk values have been produced, it was necessary to make them thicker to improve durability, thus reducing the oxygen supply to the cornea. Furthermore, these lenses were subject to lens deposits, which caused a decline in visual performance.

Disposable soft contact lenses made from high-water-content materials with consistently high performance (developed in the United States) were introduced into the Japanese market in 1991. Compared with hard contact lenses, these newer disposable soft contact lenses provide a greater degree of comfort, are safer, and do not cause conjunctival injection associated with 3 and 9 o'clock staining. It seems likely that they will become the leading type of contact lens used in Japan in the future. Japanese ophthalmologists who have been wary of extended-wear lenses in the past are expected to prescribe soft contact lenses more often in the future, due to the emergence of the disposable types of soft contact lenses.

Daily-replacement disposable soft contact lenses have been available in Japan since 1995. Because the lenses are worn once and discarded each day, they are ideal in terms of comfort and safety; their only drawback is higher cost.

DISPOSABLE EXTENDED-WEAR SOFT CONTACT LENSES

Of the three types of disposable extended-wear soft contact lenses sold in the United States (Table 7.1), the SeeQuence 2 is a low-water-content lens, whereas the ACUVUE and NewVues lenses are high-water-content lenses. According to a report by Holden and Mertz (1984), extended-wear use is comparatively safe as long as the oxygen transmissibility (*Dk/L*) value of the lens is 34 or greater. Although a few lenses meet this criterion, most extended-wear lenses still present difficulties due to their low water content.

Disposable extended-wear soft contact lenses are supplied without a case to discourage storage or reuse once they are removed from the eye. Nevertheless, complications stemming from improper usage have been reported (Cohen et al. 1991; Maguen et al. 1992; Poggio et al. 1989, 1993; Schein et al. 1989, 1994). Patients have been known to store their lenses in tap water and then put them back into the eye. Also, there are many reports of *Acanthamoeba* infection associated with improper storage in contaminated tap water, storage cases, and cleaning and storage solutions.

FREQUENT-REPLACEMENT DISPOSABLE
SOFT CONTACT LENSES

Frequent-replacement lens systems, in which the lenses are regularly replaced every 2–12 weeks, are made from the same materials as are disposable extended-wear soft contact lenses. Frequent-replacement lenses, however, are removed from the eye and

Table 7.1 Disposable Extended-Wear Soft Contact Lenses

Factor	ACUVUE	NewVues	SeeQuence	SeeQuence 2
Manufacturer	Johnson & Johnson (Jacksonville, FL)	CIBA Vision (Duluth, GA)	Bausch & Lomb (Rochester, NY)	Bausch & Lomb
Material	Etafilcon A	Vifilcon A	Polymacon	Polymacon
Water content (%)	58	55	38.6	38.6
Production method	Stabilized soft molding	Molding	Spincast	Spincast, lathed back
U.S. Food and Drug Administration group	Group 4	Group 4	Group 1	Group 1
Base curve (mm)	8.8, 8.4 (9.1)	8.8, 8.4	8.8	8.4, 8.7, 9.0
Diameter (mm)	14.0 (14.4)	14.0	14.0	14.0
Center thickness (–3.00 D) (mm)	0.07	0.06	0.035	0.035
Dk value[a]	28	16	8.4	8.4
Dk/L value[b]	40	27	24	24

[a] $\times 10^{-11}$ (cm^2/sec) • (ml O$_2$/ml • mm Hg).

[b] $\times 10^{-9}$ (cm/sec) • (ml O$_2$/ml • mm Hg).

cleaned periodically during the period of use and therefore usually are marketed in conjunction with a disinfection system (Table 7.2).

The Medalist lens (Bausch & Lomb) is marketed together with the ReNu disinfection system (also by Bausch & Lomb). The SUREVUE lens (Johnson & Johnson), which is 1.5 times thicker than the ACUVUE lens from the same company, is marketed in combination with OPTI-FREE disinfection solutions. The ACUVUE lens is used also as a frequent-replacement soft contact lens, although some patients have complained that the lens is so thin that they cannot distinguish between the front and back of the lens once it has been removed from the eye.

The Medalist lens is manufactured by the same spincasting and lathe-cutting method used to make the Optima FW (Bausch & Lomb) and SeeQuence 2 lenses and is believed to be an improvement over the SeeQuence disposable extended-wear soft contact lens in terms of safety and comfort. Our own clinical studies have shown fewer problems with the Medalist lens than with the SeeQuence lens, even with extended wear. Because both lenses are made from the same material and have the same thickness, we believe that the disparity is the result of differences in lens design and production.

Because frequent-replacement soft contact lenses are taken out of the eye periodically, they must be disinfected before they are worn again. In the United States, 99% of soft contact lenses are disinfected by chemical care systems. In Japan, only one chemical care system has been permitted to be sold, and that only since 1995; therefore, 90% of Japanese contact lens wearers still use heat disinfection systems. However, heat systems can deform high-water-content disposable soft contact lenses; consequently, as this type of lens has become more popular, the use of chemical care systems has increased.

Chemical care systems can be divided into those that contain hydrogen peroxide (CONSEPT [Allergan, Irvine, CA], AOSEPT [CIBA Vision], OxySept [Allergan],

Table 7.2 Frequent-Replacement Disposable Soft Contact Lenses

Factor	SUREVUE	Focus	Medalist
Manufacturer	Johnson & Johnson (Jacksonville, FL)	CIBA Vision Corp. (Duluth, GA)	Bausch & Lomb (Rochester, NY)
Material	Etafilcon A	Vifilcon A	Polymacon
Water content (%)	58	55	38.6
Production method	Stabilized soft molding	Molding	Spincast, lathed back
U.S. Food and Drug Administration group	Group 4	Group 4	Group 1
Base curve (mm)	8.8, 8.4 (+lens 9.1)	8.6, 8.9	8.4, 8.7, 9.0
Diameter (mm)	14.0 (+lens 14.4)	14.0	14.0
Center thickness (−3.00 D) (mm)	0.105	0.10	0.035
Dk value[a]	28	16	8.4
Dk/L value[b]	26.7	16	24
Replacement	2 wks	1 mo	1, 2, or 3 mos
Disinfection method	Chemical and oxidation	Chemical and oxidation	Heat, chemical, and oxidation

[a] $\times 10^{-11}$ (cm^2/sec) • (ml O$_2$/ml • mm Hg).
[b] $\times 10^{-9}$ (cm/sec) • (ml O$_2$/ml • mm Hg).

Table 7.3 Chemical Care Systems

Hydrogen peroxide (3% solution) systems
    AOSEPT (CIBA Vision, Duluth, GA)
    LENSEPT (CIBA Vision)
    MiraSept disinfecting solution (Alcon, Fort Worth, TX)
    OXYSEPT (Allergan, Irvine, CA)
    ULTRACARE (Allergan)
Systems without hydrogen peroxide (one-step solution)
    OPTI-FREE (Alcon): disinfecting agent, 0.001% polyquaternium-1
    ReNu (Bausch & Lomb, Rochester, NY): disinfecting agent, 0.00005% polyaminopropyl biguanide

etc.) and those that do not (OPTI-FREE [Alcon, Fort Worth, TX] , ReNu [Bausch & Lomb], etc.). Hydrogen peroxide systems involve two steps—disinfection with hydrogen peroxide and neutralization—and care must be taken because severe inflammation can result if the neutralizing step is neglected. Systems that do not use hydrogen peroxide require only one step and probably are somewhat safer and certainly more convenient (Lowe et al. 1992) (Table 7.3).

DAILY-REPLACEMENT DISPOSABLE SOFT CONTACT LENSES

As of this writing, two companies—Johnson & Johnson (1•DAY ACUVUE) and Bausch & Lomb (Occasions)—are marketing daily-replacement disposable soft contact lenses in the United States (Table 7.4). Concern has been expressed that pro-

Table 7.4 Daily-Replacement Disposable Soft Contact Lenses

Factor	1·DAY ACUVUE	Occasions
Manufacturer	Johnson & Johnson (Jacksonville, FL)	Bausch & Lomb (Rochester, NY)
Material	Etafilcon A	Polymacon
Water content (%)	58	38.6
Production method	Soft molding	Spincast
U.S. Food and Drug Administration group	Group 4	Group 1
Base curve (mm)	9.0	8.7
Diameter (mm)	14.2	14.0
Center thickness (–3.00 D) (mm)	0.07	0.043
Dk value[a]	28	8.4
Dk/L value[b]	40	19.5

[a] $\times 10^{-11}$ (cm^2/sec) • (ml O$_2$/ml • mm Hg).
[b] $\times 10^{-9}$ (cm/sec) • (ml O$_2$/ml • mm Hg).

duction of lenses designed to be used for only 1 day might imply inferior materials or performance, higher cost, or both. There are many advantages associated with daily-replacement disposable soft contact lenses, however, and many patients are likely to be willing to bear some increase in cost to obtain the ease of use and reduced risk of problems offered by these lenses.

The low rate of complications in daily-replacement lens wearers has been demonstrated in several studies. In 1992, we evaluated the complications of contact lens wear in 23,068 patients (45,580 eyes) in our clinics in Osaka, Japan (Hamano et al. 1994). Of these, 1,400 patients wore the ACUVUE lens on a daily-replacement schedule. The rate of corneal complications for the various types of lenses were: polymethyl methacrylate lenses, 15.8%; rigid gas-permeable lenses, 10.5%; acryl elastomer lenses, 7.2%; hydroxyethyl methacrylate lenses, 8.5%; high-water-content lenses, 4.0%; disposable extended-wear soft contact lenses, 4.9%; daily-replacement disposable soft lenses, 2.5%. Thus, the daily-replacement disposable lens wearers encountered the fewest problems.

In another study, we surveyed 402 patients (795 eyes) who wore daily-replacement disposable soft contact lenses. Among these patients were a number who previously had discontinued contact lens wear for various reasons and for whom the switch to daily-replacement disposable soft contact lenses made contact lens wear again possible. For 281 of these eyes, we had the records from the previous contact lens experience and the findings from ophthalmic examinations during the first week of daily-replacement lens wear and successive 3-month follow-up visits (Table 7.5) (Watanabe 1995). Bulbar conjunctival injection, superficial punctate keratopathy, and lid-conjunctival abnormalities, such as allergic conjunctivitis, were the most common problems with the previous lenses, whereas no abnormalities were seen in 92.6% of the eyes after the initiation of daily-replacement lens wear. Patients who had had superficial punctate keratopathy caused by rigid gas-permeable lenses showed particular improvement. Patients with tear deficiencies also appeared to benefit from the switch to the daily-replacement lenses.

Table 7.5 Change in Findings in Eyes of Contact Lens–Wearing Patients After Switching to Daily-Replacement Disposable Contact Lenses (281 Eyes)

Finding	Initial Examination (Number of Eyes)	Last Examination (Number of Eyes)	Percentage Decrease
Lid-conjunctiva abnormalities	122	15	87.7
Bulbar conjunctival injection	117	8	93.2
Corneal staining (SPK)	81	6	92.6
Corneal edema	2	0	100.0
Corneal neovascularization	12	0	100.0
Other	6	0	100.0
Total	338	29	91.4

SPK = superficial punctate keratopathy.

Note: All patients wore contact lenses of various types before switching to daily-replacement disposable lenses. The initial examination was performed before daily-replacement disposable lens wear was initiated. The last examination was performed at the most recent visit. Some eyes had more than one finding.

Source: Reprinted with permission from K Watanabe. Dry eye and contact lens wear. J Eye 1995;12:907.

STUDIES OF PROBLEMS ASSOCIATED WITH CONTACT LENS WEAR

In the past, soft contact lens wear required time-consuming lens care, including cleaning and disinfection, because the lenses were subject to the buildup of deposits with prolonged wear and the patients experienced an increased risk of giant papillary conjunctivitis and allergic conjunctivitis. Moreover, the low Dk of the lenses led to the problem of a chronic deficiency in the oxygen supply to the cornea.

With disposable soft contact lenses, many of these problems have been overcome. The oxygen tension measured on the cornea under these lenses is approximately that of hard lenses with high Dk. Moreover, because these lenses are discarded before deposits form, they do not contribute to the development of allergies. Although lens breakage and other mechanical stress-related problems are associated with these lenses because they are so thin, the frequent-disposal schedule lessens the need for long-term durability.

In Japan, soft contact lenses were thought to cause more problems than rigid gas-permeable lenses because their thickness and low water content and low Dk values resulted in poor oxygen transmission to the cornea. Additionally, when problems developed, patients tended to ignore such warning symptoms as discomfort, and the resulting delay in treatment led to worsened difficulties.

Ocular disorders associated with conventional soft contact lenses include (1) conditions associated with chronic oxygen deficiency (epithelial edema, corneal neovascularization), (2) conditions caused by allergic reactions (allergic conjunctivitis, giant papillary conjunctivitis, contact lens–related papillary conjunctivitis), (3) conditions caused by infection (corneal infiltration, corneal ulcer), and (4) conditions associated with tear deficiency (superficial punctate keratopathy). Daily-replacement or frequent-replacement disposable soft contact lenses alleviate or prevent many of these problems.

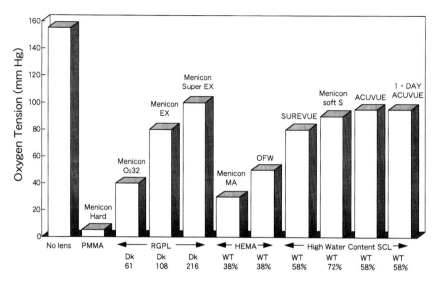

Figure 7.2 Oxygen tension on the cornea without a contact lens and with various types of rigid and soft contact lenses. (PMMA = polymethyl methacrylate lens; RGPL = rigid gas-permeable lens; HEMA = hydroxyethyl methacrylate; SCL = soft contact lens; Dk = oxygen permeability of lens material; WT = water content.)

Chronic Oxygen Deficiency

Contact lens wear decreases the supply of oxygen to the cornea and causes increased corneal thickness, decreased cell proliferation, increased lactic acid in the aqueous humor (from metabolism of glycogen), and decreased numbers of corneal nerves.

Daily-replacement and frequent-replacement disposable lenses achieve greater oxygen supply to the cornea because they are manufactured from high-water-content materials and are designed to be more mobile on the cornea. Also, deposits that might interfere with oxygen transmission are prevented by replacement of the lenses with new lenses at regular intervals.

Water Content and Oxygen Permeability

The Dk value, expressed as units $\times 10^{-11}$ (cm²/sec) • (ml O$_2$/ml • mm Hg), generally is used as the index for the oxygen permeability of a lens material. The oxygen transmissibility (Dk/L) of a given lens is derived by dividing the Dk value by the thickness of the lens in centimeters, expressed as units $\times 10^{-9}$ (cm/sec) • (ml O$_2$/ml • mm Hg). Most manufacturers provide this Dk/L value; however, because the method of measurement often differs from one company to another, direct comparison of Dk/L values is difficult.

We used a platinum microelectrode (Hamano et al. 1984; 1986a, b) to measure the oxygen tension on the normal cornea with no contact lens as well as on corneas wearing various types of contact lenses (Figure 7.2). We found that the oxygen tension on the cornea under a low-water-content soft contact lens is only one-third to one-fifth that of a normal eye without a lens. With a high-water-content soft contact lens, however, the oxygen tension was in the range of two-thirds that of a normal, non–lens-wearing eye. We also observed a correlation between the Dk/L value and the oxygen partial pressure at the corneal surface; for the lenses tested, the partial pressures of oxygen were 95 mm

Hg for the ACUVUE lens, with a Dk/L = 40×10^{-9}; 85 mm Hg for the SUREVUE lens, with a Dk/L = 27×10^{-9}; 76 mm Hg for the NewVues lens, with a Dk/L = 27×10^{-9}; and 50 mm Hg for the Optima FW lens, with a Dk/L = 24×10^{-9}.

Lens Design

Contact lens design varies greatly, depending on the manufacturer and method of production, and the design has a major impact on the safety and performance of the lens. For example, lens thickness is important, not only centrally but also peripherally; lenses that are very thin at the center must be somewhat thicker in the periphery to obtain proper movement of the lens on the cornea. Now that disposable soft contact lenses have become available at a relatively low cost per unit, patients may wonder why previous soft contact lenses were so expensive.

The main reason is that newer methods of production have allowed the recent decreases in price. Previously, lathe-cutting machines with diamond tools were used, and costs were high because the machines were expensive and production was time consuming. In contrast, ACUVUE and NewVues lenses are made by the molding method, in which material is sandwiched from above and below and, essentially, stamped into shape. This lowers the cost because large quantities of lenses can be produced with a high degree of precision. The spincast method used to make the SeeQuence lens also is associated with low production costs.

We used videokeratography (TMS-1, Tomey, Nagoya, Japan) to evaluate contact lens correction and fitting by measuring the topography of the soft contact lens on the eye (Watanabe et al. 1992). Specifically, we applied differential mapping to determine the refractive power distribution of the soft contact lenses on the cornea. We examined three different types of soft contact lenses that varied in manufacturing method and design (Figure 7.3) in the eyes of myopic patients, and the subjective evaluations of the patients, including comfort and vision, were correlated with the numeric indexes produced by the videokeratoscope (Table 7.6). The surface regularity index (SRI) and the surface asymmetry index (SAI), two indexes that numerically express visual potential in terms of corneal shape, appeared to correlate well with subjective visual acuity. Differential surface mapping comparing corneal contours with and without a contact lens displayed the refractive power distribution of both the contact lens and the tear layer (Figure 7.4). The ACUVUE lens, with a refractive power of approximately –5 D, provided uniform power distribution on the central cornea; the patients' subjective evaluations showed that this was the most comfortable lens and provided the best vision. The Optima FW lens also provided sufficient power and uniform refraction over the entire surface of the lens. The SeeQuence lens had a refractive power of –4 to –5 D, but the power dropped to approximately –3 D at the periphery. This correlated with the subjective finding of decreased visual acuity during blinking due to lens movement. In all, this approach provides useful information about lens surface topography that may be valuable in improving soft contact lens design.

Lens Deposits

Deposits form on contact lenses even with proper, regular care. These deposits are composed of a film of protein, calcium, lipid, and bacterial by-products. In 1985, the U.S. Food and Drug Administration (FDA) classified soft contact lenses into four

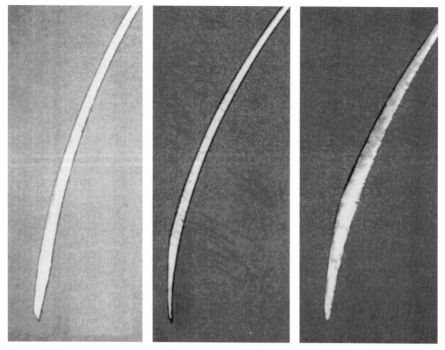

Figure 7.3 Cross-sections of three soft contact lenses produced by different methods. Left to right: stabilized soft molding (ACUVUE, Johnson & Johnson, Jacksonville, FL); spincast (See-Quence, Bausch & Lomb, Rochester, NY); spincast lathed (Optima FW, Bausch & Lomb).

Table 7.6 Videokeratographic Evaluation of Cornea–Contact Lens Topography in Eyes With and Without Contact Lenses

Topographic Index	No Contact Lens	ACUVUE (Johnson & Johnson, Jacksonville, FL)	SeeQuence (Bausch & Lomb, Rochester, NY)	Optima FW (Bausch & Lomb)
SRI	0.57 ± 0.21	0.46 ± 0.10	0.63 ± 0.29	0.54 ± 0.07
SAI	0.39 ± 0.13	0.34 ± 0.07	0.56 ± 0.13	0.46 ± 0.18

SRI = surface regularity index; SAI = surface asymmetry index.
Note: These indexes are numeric values derived from topography analysis using the TMS-1 videokeratoscope (Tomey, Nagoya, Japan). The lower the number, the more regular the surface and the greater the potential for good visual acuity. $N = 10$ eyes in each group. Values are mean ± standard deviation.
Source: Reprinted with permission from K Watanabe, N Maeda, H Hamano, et al. Evaluation of soft contact lenses using TMS-1. J Jpn Contact Lens Soc 1992;34:58.

groups based on material and water content: group 1, low water content (<50% H_2O), nonionic polymers; group 2, high water content (>50% H_2O), nonionic polymers; group 3, low water content (<50% H_2O), ionic polymers; and group 4, high water content (>50% H_2O), ionic polymers.

High-water-content polymer lenses generally are associated with greater deposit formation than are low-water-content polymer lenses. Furthermore, ionic polymers are subject to greater deposit formation than are nonionic polymers. Thus, the soft

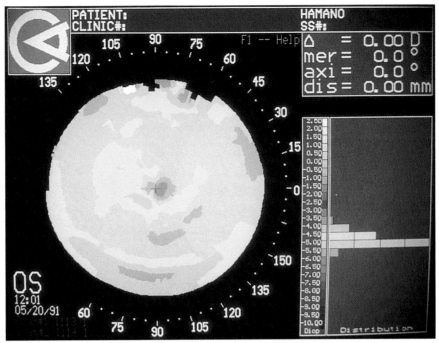

A

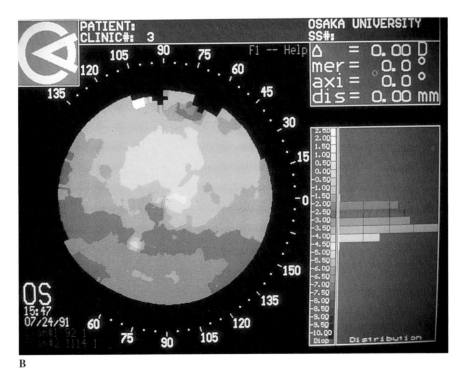

B

Figure 7.4 Topographic analysis of three different soft contact lenses on the cornea using the TMS-1 videokeratoscope (Tomey, Nagoya, Japan). A. ACUVUE (Johnson & Johnson, Jacksonville, FL). B. SeeQuence (Bausch & Lomb, Rochester, NY).

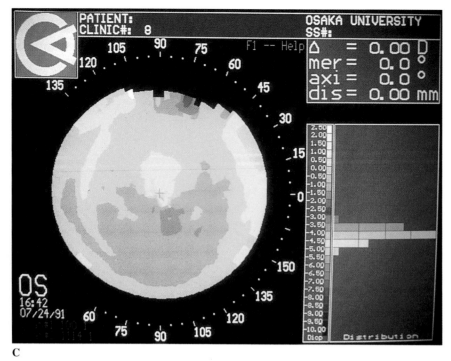

C

Figure 7.4 (*continued*) C. Optima FW (Bausch & Lomb).

contact lenses in group 4 should be used for shorter rather than longer periods of time before they are replaced.

We also used videokeratography to investigate topographic differences between worn and unworn, low-water-content, nonionic polymer soft contact lenses (FDA group 1) on 12 eyes of 11 patients who had worn soft contact lenses for more than 1 year and who showed a decrease in best-corrected visual acuity (Hamano et al. 1992). An irregular distribution of refractive powers was observed in 10 of the 12 eyes with the old lens in place; mean (± standard deviation) SRI for this group of eyes was 2.38 ± 1.72, and mean (± standard deviation) SAI was 1.27 ± 0.60. When new lenses were placed on these eyes, the distribution of powers was more regular, with a mean SRI of 0.51 ± 0.16 and a mean SAI of 0.41 ± 0.13. The differences between the values for the worn and new lenses were significant. Thus, we conclude that when this type of contact lens is worn over a long period of time, the lens surface may become asymmetric as a result of the formation of lens deposits, leading to a decline in best-corrected visual acuity.

Conjunctival Allergic Reactions

The incidence of giant papillary conjunctivitis (Allansmith et al. 1977) appears to be on the rise in Japan, corresponding to the increased number of contact lens wearers. Lens deposits are thought to be a contributing factor to the development of this disorder (Donshik and Ballow 1983; Richard et al. 1992). With daily-replacement or frequent-replacement disposable soft contact lens systems, however, each lens is worn for only a short period of time, minimizing the opportunity for deposits to build up. Based on a clinical trial that involved scanning electron microscopic observation of the surface of used lenses (Figure 7.5), we concluded that the reduced risk of

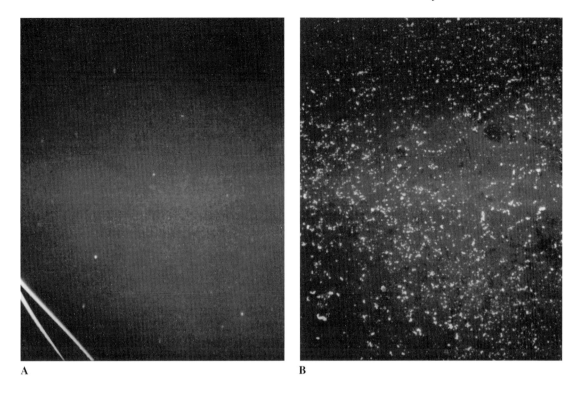

A   B

Figure 7.5 Scanning electron microscopy of the surface of soft contact lenses. A. Lens never worn. B. Normal eye; lens worn 1 week. C. Patient with giant papillary conjunctivitis; lens worn 1 week.

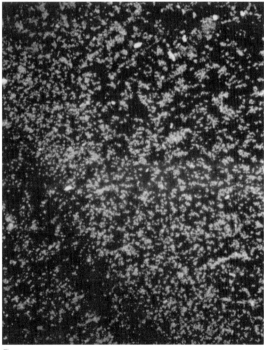

C

deposit buildup with disposable lenses made these lenses safer for use in patients with giant papillary conjunctivitis (Watanabe et al. 1993).

Infections

Acanthamoeba infection is one of the most severe complications associated with contact lens wear. Although this problem has been seen occasionally in patients who use chemical disinfectants, it is much more common among those who use homemade saline solutions to clean and store their lenses. In 1989, the FDA restricted the sale of salt tablets and issued a notice to ophthalmologists warning against the use of homemade saline cleaning solutions. Since then, the incidence of *Acanthamoeba* infection has declined somewhat, but sporadic cases still occur.

When used properly, disposable lenses require little care and reduce the risk of infection due to bacteria or *Acanthamoeba*. It must be noted, however, that there have been reports of *Acanthamoeba* infection in patients who reuse disposable lenses that should have been discarded. Thus, patient education and compliance are essential for appropriate use and storage of lenses, both of which are major factors in the safety of contact lens wear.

Tear Deficiency

Superficial punctate keratopathy occurs frequently in patients with reduced tear production, even in those not using contact lenses. Thus, the use of contact lenses in patients with severe tear deficiency is difficult or impossible, but problems also are seen commonly in patients with only mild dry eyes.

The normal volume of tears is between 1 and 1.6 µl, with surface evaporation dissipating 6% of the secreted volume. Contact lens wear causes an increase in evaporation from the surface of the eye. In normal eyes, this change in the amount of evaporation with contact lens use still allows the tear volume to remain within the normal range. In eyes that are deficient in tears, however, rigid gas-permeable lenses can lead to localized drying of the cornea, characterized by staining at the 3 and 9 o'clock locations, and patient complaints of ocular irritation and discomfort.

The amount of tear secretion declines one-fifth to one-tenth during sleep. Therefore, when disposable extended-wear soft contact lenses are worn overnight, superficial punctate keratopathy can occur due to drying, even in normal eyes, but particularly in eyes with mild tear deficiency. In virtually all cases, the keratopathy is limited to the inferior cornea and usually disappears with frequent application of artificial tear solution. To prevent the sensation of dryness on awakening often experienced with continuous use of disposable extended-wear soft contact lenses, we encourage patients to apply artificial tear solutions on a regular basis on waking, even in the middle of the night. Our experience is that keeping a bottle of artificial tears at the bedside and applying them whenever the patient wakens sufficiently to open his or her eyes reduces the occurrence of superficial punctate keratopathy. If this approach is not successful, however, daily-replacement disposable soft contact lenses, frequent-replacement soft contact lenses, or other types of soft lenses may eliminate the problem.

REFERENCES

Allansmith MR, Dorb DR, Greiner JV, et al. Giant papillary conjunctivitis in contact lens wearers. Am J Ophthalmol 1977;83:697.

Cohen EJ, Gonzalez C, Leavitt KG, et al. Corneal ulcers associated with contact lenses including experience with disposable lenses. CLAO J 1991;17:173.

Donshik PC, Ballow M. Tear immunoglobulins in giant papillary conjunctivitis induced by contact lenses. Am J Ophthalmol 1983;96:460.

Hamano H, Hamano T, Hamano T, et al. Comparison between old and new soft contact lenses' surface shape during wear. J Jpn Contact Lens Soc 1992;34:53.

Hamano H, Mikami M, Mohri H, Mitsunaga S. Measurement of oxygen partial pressure at the rabbit cornea under various types of contact lenses. J Jpn Contact Lens Soc 1984;26:295.

Hamano H, Mikami M, Mohri H, et al. Measurement of oxygen tension in anterior ocular segments by a platinum microelectrode. I. Preliminary experiments in vitro system. J Jpn Contact Lens Soc 1986a;28:47.

Hamano H, Mikami M, Mohri H, et al. Measurement of oxygen tension in anterior ocular segments by a platinum microelectrode. II. In vivo measurement of oxygen tension on rabbit and human cornea under various gas permeable hard contact lenses. J Jpn Contact Lens Soc 1986b;28:51.

Hamano H, Watanabe K, Hamano T, et al. A study of complications induced by conventional and disposable contact lenses. CLAO J 1994;20:103.

Holden BA, Mertz GW. Critical oxygen levels to avoid corneal edema for daily and extended wear contact lenses. Invest Ophthalmol Vis Sci 1984;25:1161.

Lowe R, Vallas V, Brennan N. Comparative efficacy of contact lens disinfection solutions. CLAO J 1992;18:34.

Maguen E, Rosner I, Caroline P, et al. A retrospective study of disposable extended wear lenses in 100 patients: year 2. CLAO J 1992;18:229.

Poggio EC, Abelson M. Complications and symptoms in disposable extended wear lenses compared with conventional soft daily wear and soft extended wear lenses. CLAO J 1993;19:31.

Poggio EC, Glynn RJ, Schein OD, et al. The incidence of ulcerative keratitis among users of daily wear and extended wear soft contact lenses. N Engl J Med 1989;321:779.

Richard NR, Anderson JA, Tasevska ZG, Binder PS. Evaluation of tear protein deposits on contact lenses from patients with and without giant papillary conjunctivitis. CLAO J 1992;18:143.

Schein OD, Buehler PO, Stamler JF, et al. The impact of overnight wear on the risk of contact lens associated ulcerative keratitis. Arch Ophthalmol 1994;112:186.

Schein OD, Glynn RJ, Poggio EC, et al. The relative risk of ulcerative keratitis among users of daily wear and extended wear soft contact lenses. A case control study. N Engl J Med 1989;321:773.

Watanabe K. Dry eye and contact lens wear. J Eye 1995;12:907.

Watanabe K, Kida K, Ohashi Y, et al. Disposable extended-wear soft contact lenses for giant papillary conjunctivitis. J Jpn Contact Lens Soc 1993;35:126.

Watanabe K, Maeda N, Hamano H, Manabe R. Evaluation of soft contact lenses using TMS-1. J Jpn Contact Lens Soc 1992;34:58.

8

Safety of Daily-Disposable Contact Lenses: A Study of Corneal Complications*

Hikaru Hamano

During the 1990s, many changes in contact lens wear have resulted from the development of new types of lenses, including the most recent innovation: daily-disposable lenses. In concert with these changes in lens materials, manufacturing processes, and wear patterns, the types and incidences of complications related to contact lens wear also have changed.

Conventional daily-wear soft contact lenses used as extended-wear lenses generally are associated with a higher incidence of complications than are the same lenses used on a daily-wear schedule (Poggio et al. 1989; Schein et al. 1989; Buehler et al. 1992; Matthews et al. 1992; Stapleton et al. 1992; Poggio and Abelson 1993). Other studies have found that complication rates for disposable extended-wear lenses are not markedly different from the rates for conventional soft lenses used on an extended-wear schedule (Laibson et al. 1993; Poggio and Abelson 1993). However, the relative risk for corneal ulcers with disposable extended-wear lenses has been reported to range from approximately 7 to 15 times that for conventional daily-wear soft lenses (Buehler et al. 1992; Matthews et al. 1992).

The results of studies of contact lens wear complications depend not only on the methodology used but also on the type of institution in which the study is carried out. One would expect the results of a clinical study at a university hospital to differ from the results of studies involving patients in private practice because the characteristics of the two populations are different. Furthermore, as in all controlled studies, the manner of selection of the control population also can affect results. In addition, the distribution of types of lenses worn differs from one country to another (e.g., in the early 1990s, daily-wear rigid gas-permeable lenses predominated in Japan, whereas in the United States, soft lenses were more popular).

In 1993, we undertook a large-scale evaluation of complications caused by contact lens wear in our private-practice patients in Osaka, Japan (Hamano et al. 1994). We examined the types of lenses prescribed, including hard and soft lenses; the patterns of wear, including conventional daily wear, extended wear, and daily-dispos-

---

*Parts of this chapter were adapted with permission from H Hamano, K Watanabe, T Hamano, et al. A study of the complications induced by conventional and disposable contact lenses. CLAO J 1994;20:103.

Table 8.1 Classification of Contact Lenses

Contact Lens	Wearing Schedule	Major Brand (Manufacturer)	Water Content (%)	Dk
Hard				
PMMA	Daily	Menicon Hard (Menicon, Nagoya, Japan)	—	—
RGP	Daily	Low Dk: Menicon O$_2$	—	13
		Mid Dk: Menicon O$_2$-32	—	61
		High Dk: Menicon EX, Super EX (all by Menicon)	—	>100
Soft				
Elastomer	Daily	SOPHINA (Ricky, Tokyo, Japan)	—	34
HEMA	Daily	Menicon Soft MA (Menicon) Optima FW (Bausch & Lomb, Rochester, NY)	38	9.5–13.0
High-water-content	Daily	Menicon Soft 72 (Menicon)	72	51
Weekly-disposable	Extended	ACUVUE (Johnson & Johnson, Jacksonville, FL)	58	28
Daily-disposable	Daily	1•DAY ACUVUE (Johnson & Johnson)*	58	28

PMMA = polymethyl methacrylate; RGP = rigid gas-permeable; elastomer = acryl elastomer; HEMA = hydroxyethyl methacrylate; Dk = oxygen permeability [$\times 10^{-11}$ (cm^2/sec) • (ml O$_2$/ml • mm Hg)].
*Not commercially available in Japan at the time of the study.
Source: Reprinted with permission from H Hamano, K Watanabe, T Hamano, et al. A study of the complications induced by conventional and disposable contact lenses. CLAO J 1994;20:103.

able wear; and the types and incidence of various corneal findings in the total population and in each group of lens wearers.

CONTACT LENSES

The types of contact lenses worn by patients in this study are shown in Table 8.1. Hard lenses included polymethyl methacrylate (PMMA) and rigid gas-permeable lenses. Soft lenses included five types of lenses: three daily-wear lenses (an acryl elastomer–based lens with 0% water content; a 38% low-water-content, hydroxyethyl methacrylate [HEMA]–based lens; and a 72% high-water-content, dimethyl acrylamide–based lens) and two types of disposable lenses. One disposable lens is designed for extended wear lasting up to 1 week, and the other is used for only 1 day and then is discarded.

Three of these types of lenses—the high-water-content lens, the weekly-disposable lens, and the daily-disposable lens—have been prescribed at our clinics only since 1992. At the time of this study, daily-disposable lenses were not commercially available and were therefore prescribed on an investigational basis.

PATIENTS

The contact lens patients who participated in the study were examined between December 1992 and February 1993 at one of six eye clinics in Osaka, Japan. Table

Table 8.2 Sex and Age Distribution of Patients in the Study Population

Classification	All Patients (%) (n = 23,068)		Patients with Complications (%) (n = 2,693)	
Sex				
Male	6,205	(26.9)	600	(22.3)
Female	16,863	(73.1)	2,093	(77.7)
Age (yrs)				
≤9	4	(<0.1)	3	(0.1)
10–19	2,252	(9.8)	236	(8.8)
20–29	10,556	(45.7)	1,300	(48.2)
30–39	5,917	(25.7)	671	(25.0)
40–49	3,229	(14.0)	347	(12.9)
50–59	845	(3.7)	108	(4.0)
60–69	217	(0.9)	27	(1.0)
≥70	48	(0.2)	1	(<0.1)

Source: Reprinted with permission from H Hamano, K Watanabe, T Hamano, et al. A study of the complications induced by conventional and disposable contact lenses. CLAO J 1994;20:103.

8.2 shows the sex and age distributions of the patients. The study was designed to last for 3 months because, in Japan, wearers of disposable lenses are scheduled for an office visit at least once every 3 months for a routine examination and to receive a new supply of lenses.

COMPLICATIONS

Before the study began, the prospective examining ophthalmologists were given a classification of corneal findings to use as a guide in making sketches in the patients' records (Figure 8.1). At the end of the study, we collated the numbers and types of corneal problems recorded for each patient. Chart information frequently did not specify whether conjunctivitis was caused by contact lens wear, seasonal allergies, or a drug reaction; consequently, this disease category was excluded from the study.

The incidence of complications was calculated by using as the denominator the total number of eyes wearing contact lenses in the study population. Statistical significance was determined by using a two-tailed test based on the normal distribution.

Incidence of Complications in All Patients

During the 3-month period of study, 23,068 patients (45,580 eyes) were examined at the six clinics. Corneal complications related to contact lens wear were found in nearly 10% of the eyes (2,693 patients, 4,363 eyes; Table 8.3).

Incidence of Complications for Various Types of Contact Lenses

The incidence of corneal complications in relation to each type of contact lens is shown in Table 8.3. The percentage of eyes with complications was highest for the

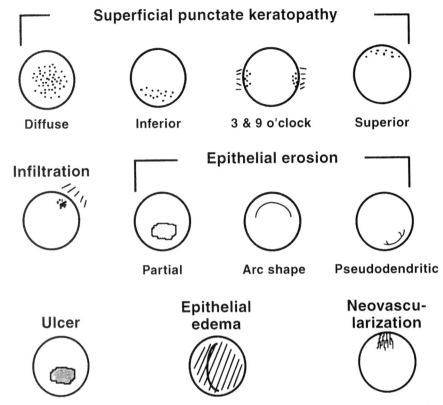

Figure 8.1 Classification of corneal findings associated with contact lens wear. (Reprinted with permission from H Hamano, K Watanabe, T Hamano, et al. A study of the complications induced by conventional and disposable contact lenses. CLAO J 1994;20:103.)

Table 8.3 Incidence of Complications with Various Types of Contact Lenses

| Contact Lens | Number of Eyes | | Incidence* (%) (95% CI) |
	All Patients (%)	Patients with Complications (%)	
Hard			
PMMA	2,267 (5.0)	358 (8.2)	15.8 (14.3–17.3%)
RGP	30,459 (66.8)	3,191 (73.1)	10.5 (10.2–10.8%)
Soft			
Elastomer	124 (0.3)	9 (0.2)	7.2 (2.7–11.7%)
HEMA	6,261 (13.7)	534 (12.2)	8.5 (7.8–9.2%)
High-water-content	2,591 (5.7)	103 (2.4)	4.0 (3.6–4.4%)
Weekly-disposable	2,985 (6.5)	146 (3.3)	4.9 (4.1–5.7%)
Daily-disposable	893 (2.0)	22 (0.5)	2.5 (1.5–3.5%)
Total	45,580 (100.0)	4,363 (100.0)	9.6

CI = confidence interval; PMMA = polymethyl methacrylate; RGP = rigid gas-permeable; elastomer = acryl elastomer; HEMA = hydroxyethyl methacrylate.
*The number of eyes with complications divided by total number of eyes wearing that type of lens.
Source: Reprinted with permission from H Hamano, K Watanabe, T Hamano, et al. A study of the complications induced by conventional and disposable contact lenses. CLAO J 1994;20:103.

Table 8.4 Probability Values (P) for Statistical Significance of Incidence Rates of Complications

Contact Lens	PMMA	RGP	Elasto-mer	HEMA	High-Water-Content	Weekly-Disposable	Daily-Disposable
PMMA		—	—	—	—	—	—
RGP	<.000001		—	—	—	—	—
Elastomer	.00906	.2380*		—	—	—	—
HEMA	<.000001	<.000001	.6030*		—	—	—
High-water-content	<.000001	<.000001	.0750*	<.000001		—	—
Weekly-disposable	<.000001	<.000001	.2502*	<.000001	.1336*		—
Daily-disposable	<.000001	<.000001	.00328	<.000001	.03236	.00270	

PMMA = polymethyl methacrylate; RGP = rigid gas-permeable; elastomer = acryl elastomer; HEMA = hydroxyethyl methacrylate.
*Not statistically significant.
Note: P <.05 indicates statistical significance.
Source: Reprinted with permission from H Hamano, K Watanabe, T Hamano, et al. A study of the complications induced by conventional and disposable contact lenses. CLAO J 1994;20:103.

PMMA hard lens wearers and lowest for the daily-disposable soft lens wearers. As shown in Table 8.4, the rate for the PMMA hard lenses was significantly higher than was the rate for any other lens and, similarly, the rate for the daily-disposable lenses was significantly lower than was the rate for any other lens.

The rate of complications with rigid gas-permeable lenses was significantly higher than the rates for the low-water-content HEMA lens and the three high-water-content lenses. Also, the rate for the low-water-content lens was significantly higher than were the rates for the three high-water-content lenses. Because of the small number of eyes using acryl elastomer lenses, the confidence interval was large, and the difference in incidence rates reached statistical significance only in comparison with the PMMA hard lenses and the daily-disposable soft lenses.

Corneal Findings

Table 8.5 shows the types of complications observed and the numbers and percentages of eyes affected by each type of corneal finding. The most common finding was superficial punctate keratopathy, regardless of the type of contact lens worn. In particular, 10.2% of eyes wearing PMMA hard lenses showed diffuse superficial punctate keratopathy, which was the basis for this group's having the highest incidence rate of corneal complications among all the lens groups. It is well known that this problem is related to corneal oxygen deficiency caused by these lenses.

Because of the high oxygen permeability of the rigid gas-permeable lens, the incidence of diffuse superficial punctate keratopathy in this group was less than one-half that of the PMMA lens group. The incidence of 3 and 9 o'clock staining was higher for the rigid gas-permeable lens group than for the PMMA lens group, how-

Table 8.5 Numbers of Eyes with Various Types of Contact Lens–Induced Corneal Complications

Contact lens	Superficial Punctate Keratopathy				
	Diffuse	**Inferior**	**3 and 9 O'clock**	**Superior**	**Infiltrate**
Hard					
PMMA (*n* = 2,267)	232 (10.2%)	22 (1.0%)	58 (2.6%)	2 (0.1%)	9 (0.4%)
RGP (*n* = 30,459)	1,267 (4.1%)	273 (0.9%)	1,325 (4.4%)	19 (<0.1%)	78 (0.2%)
Soft					
Elastomer (*n* = 124)	2 (1.6%)	5 (4.0%)	0	1 (0.8%)	1 (0.8%)
HEMA (*n* = 6,261)	218 (3.5%)	162 (2.6%)	4 (0.1%)	80 (1.3%)	24 (0.4%)
High-water-content (*n* = 2,591)	44 (1.7%)	42 (1.6%)	0	4 (0.2%)	1 (<0.1%)
Weekly-disposable (*n* = 2,985)	38 (1.3%)	95 (3.2%)	0	5 (0.2%)	4 (0.1%)
Daily-disposable (*n* = 893)	8 (0.9%)	13 (1.4%)	0	0	1 (0.1%)

n = number of eyes wearing that type of contact lens; PMMA = polymethyl methacrylate; RGP = rigid gas-permeable; elastomer = acryl elastomer; HEMA = hydroxyethyl methacrylate.
Source: Reprinted with permission from H Hamano, K Watanabe, T Hamano, et al. A study of the complications induced by conventional and disposable contact lenses. CLAO J 1994;20:103.

ever. It has been suggested that this staining is caused by a factor not directly re-lated to the oxygen permeability of the lens material.

Among the soft lenses, the low-water-content lens wearers more often showed diffuse superficial punctate keratopathy than inferiorly located disease, whereas the reverse was true for the weekly-disposable lens wearers, in whom this type of ker-atopathy usually was located inferior to the pupillary area. In contrast, the distribu-tion of superficial punctate keratopathy by location was approximately equal in wearers of high-water-content lenses and daily-disposable lenses.

Corneal infiltrates, erosions, and edema were rare or nonexistent in all lens groups. Neovascularization was seen almost exclusively in those wearing the low-water-content HEMA lenses.

No corneal ulcers were observed in this study. Based on our previous large-scale study (Hamano et al. 1988), one would expect to find one or two corneal ulcers in such a large number of patients wearing hard lenses (either PMMA or rigid gas-permeable) or low-water-content HEMA soft lenses. We confirmed, however, that the absence of corneal ulcers was possible, using the test for probability for Poisson distribution.

SAFETY OF VARIOUS TYPES OF CONTACT LENSES

Conventional Soft Lenses

The incidence of complications was significantly higher for the daily-wear, low-water-content HEMA lenses than for the daily-wear, high-water-content lenses (see Tables 8.3 and 8.4). In our study, however, the high-water-content lenses were used for less than 1 year in all cases because we began to prescribe these lenses only in 1992, whereas the low-water-content lenses were used for 1 year or more (in some cases more than 3 years) by more than half the patients in this group (Table 8.6). Although the daily-wear cleaning and sterilization procedures were the same for both of these types of lenses, the difference in incidence of complications may have been related to the differences in lens age and problems, such as lens deposits, that develop with increasing lens age.

	Epithelial Erosion					
Partial	**Arcuate**	**Pseudodendritic**	**Ulcer**	**Epithelial Edema**	**Neovascularization**	**Other**
15 (0.7%)	3 (0.1%)	2 (0.1%)	0	14 (0.6%)	2 (0.1%)	8 (0.4%)
192 (0.6%)	54 (0.2%)	1 (<0.1%)	0	2 (<0.1%)	2 (<0.1%)	22 (<0.1%)
1 (0.8%)	0	0	0	1 (0.8%)	0	0
31 (0.5%)	2 (<0.1%)	0	0	2 (<0.1%)	51 (0.8%)	3 (<0.1%)
8 (0.3%)	1 (<0.1%)	0	0	0	2 (<0.1%)	1 (<0.1%)
3 (0.1%)	0	0	0	0	0	0
0	0	0	0	0	0	0

Disposable Extended-Wear Lenses

Although the weekly-disposable lens is worn on an extended-wear schedule, the incidence of complications in this group of patients was lower than the incidence in those using the daily-wear low-water-content HEMA lens. There was, however, no significant difference compared with the incidence in the daily-wear high-water-content lens wearers. These results, and the absence of corneal ulcers, differ markedly from those reported by investigators in other countries (Buehler et al. 1992; Matthews et al. 1992).

Until recently, the daily-wear rigid gas-permeable lens was the most common type of lens used in Japan, and most ophthalmologists in Japan have been wary of prescribing extended-wear soft lenses. In our study, the prescribing ophthalmologists were instructed to provide extended-wear lenses only for patients who were known to have a high level of compliance. Furthermore, in Japan, disposable lenses are supplied only to patients who agree to return for a follow-up examination every 3 months. We believe that strict guidelines such as these help to prevent serious corneal complications with extended-wear contact lens use.

Daily-Disposable Lenses

Although the daily-disposable lens and the weekly-disposable lens are actually the same contact lens, the incidence of complications was 2.5% for the daily-disposable and roughly double that for the weekly-disposable lens. These lenses have a high oxygen permeability, but oxygen deprivation to the cornea cannot be avoided during sleep, and this problem is exacerbated by overnight lens wear, probably leading to the increased rate of complications seen with the extended-wear schedule.

In our previous study of the corneal endothelium in the presence of disposable lenses (Hamano et al. 1993), there were no endothelial changes with open eyelids. Blebs were seen to form after 20 minutes of eyelid closure, however (see Chapter 2,

Table 8.6 Duration of Use of Conventional Daily-Wear Soft Lenses

Contact Lens	<1 Year	1–2 Years	2–3 Years	>3 Years	Unknown
HEMA (n = 534)	194 (36.3%)	143 (26.8%)	78 (14.6%)	73 (13.7%)	46 (8.6%)
High-water-content (n = 103)	103 (100%)	—	—	—	—

n = number of eyes wearing that type of contact lens; HEMA = hydroxyethyl methacrylate.
Source: Reprinted with permission from H Hamano, K Watanabe, T Hamano, et al. A study of the complications induced by conventional and disposable contact lenses. CLAO J 1994;20:103.

Figures 2.6 and 2.7). Sakamoto et al. (1991) also have shown that overnight corneal swelling during extended wear with disposable lenses was 10%, which is significantly higher than that of an eye with no lens or an eye wearing a high-oxygen-permeability rigid gas-permeable lens overnight (see Chapter 2, Figures 2.8 and 2.9). Furthermore, Tsubota and Yamada (1992) reported that corneal epithelial cells become enlarged with extended-wear use of disposable lenses. These findings support the hypothesis that, despite the high oxygen permeability of the disposable lens, the cornea still undergoes marked physiologic stress with eyelid closure over the lens.

One approach to avoiding these physiologic effects with extended-wear use would be the daily-wear disposable lens, which is not worn overnight and is discarded after each day's wear. Theoretically, this type of lens should be ideal for minimizing corneal complications. The results of our large-scale 1994 study, as well as those of Solomon et al. (1996), appear to provide statistical confirmation of the clinical usefulness of the daily-disposable system.

LONG-TERM CONTINUATION OF DAILY-DISPOSABLE CONTACT LENS WEAR

During the 18-month period between July 1992 and December 1993, we prescribed daily-disposable contact lenses for a total of 1,048 patients (2,080 eyes). By the end of 1994, 567 patients (1,126 eyes) had continued to use these daily-disposable lenses for at least 5 days a week for a minimum of 1 year (Hamano et al. 1995). Thus, 54.1% of patients for whom these lenses were prescribed continued to use them.

Although the continuation of lens wear did not differ by sex, there were marked differences among the various age groups. As Figure 8.2 demonstrates, the rate of continuation of daily-disposable lens use increased with increasing age, ranging from 26.9% among teenagers to 67.9% among patients in their 40s, with further increases to 76.9% among patients in their 50s and 100% of those 60 or older (to be sure, a very small group).

When we analyzed this group in terms of refractive error, we found that in the initial group of 2,080 eyes, 14 were hyperopic, and the remainder were myopic, with refractive errors ranging from 0.5 to 9.0 D of myopia (Figure 8.3). The largest groups fell into the 2- to 4-D range. It is apparent from Figures 8.3 and 8.4 that patients with higher amounts of myopia were more likely to continue disposable contact lens wear. Whereas only 46.2% of patients with 3 or fewer diopters of myopia continued to wear these lenses, 63.2% of those with myopia of 6.5 or more diopters still were wearing daily-disposable lenses after 1 year. Thus, it appears that patients with a greater need for visual correction find the use of daily-disposable contact lenses more appealing.

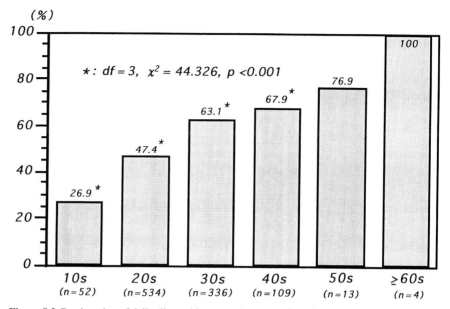

Figure 8.2 Continuation of daily-disposable contact lens wear for at least 1 year among various age groups. A total of 1,048 patients were prescribed these lenses, and 567 patients continued to use this type of lens for at least 1 year, for an overall rate of 54.1%. The rate increases significantly with age from the teenagers (10s) to the patients in their forties (40s). (Reprinted with permission from H Hamano, T Hamano, K Watanabe, et al. A study of the patients continuing daily disposable lens wear. J Jpn Contact Lens Soc 1995;37:273.)

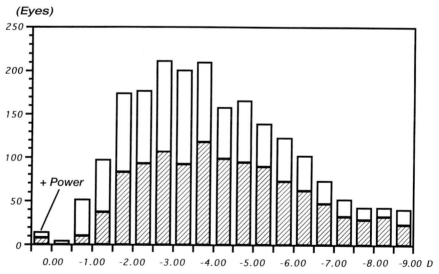

Figure 8.3 Distribution of powers of daily-disposable contact lenses prescribed for 2,080 eyes of 1,048 patients. The shaded portion of each bar indicates the number of eyes corrected with daily-disposable lenses for at least 1 year. (Reprinted with permission from H Hamano, T Hamano, K Watanabe, et al. A study of the patients continuing daily disposable lens wear. J Jpn Contact Lens Soc 1995;37:273.)

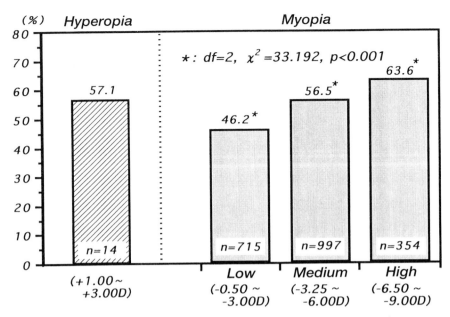

Figure 8.4 Continued daily-disposable contact lens wear for at least 1 year by contact lens power. Among the myopic patients, the rate increases significantly with increasing lens power. (Reprinted with permission from H Hamano, T Hamano, K Watanabe, et al. A study of the patients continuing daily disposable lens wear. J Jpn Contact Lens Soc 1995;37:273.)

REFERENCES

Buehler PO, Schein OD, Stamler JF, et al. The increased risk of ulcerative keratitis among disposable soft contact lens users. Arch Ophthalmol 1992;110:1555.

Hamano H, Hamano T, Hamano T, et al. Clinical evaluation of various contact lenses from the incidence of complications. J Br Contact Lens Assoc 1988;11:25.

Hamano H, Hamano T, Watanabe K, et al. A study of the patients continuing daily disposable lens wear [in Japanese]. J Jpn Contact Lens Soc 1995;37:273.

Hamano H, Watanabe K, Hamano T, et al. A study of the complications induced by conventional and disposable contact lenses. CLAO J 1994;20:103.

Hamano H, Watanabe K, Mitsunaga S. Observation of corneal endothelial response to hydrogel lenses by non-contact specular microscope (TOPCON SP1000) [in Japanese]. J Jpn Contact Lens Soc 1993;35:140.

Laibson PR, Cohen EJ, Rajpal RK. Corneal ulcers related to contact lenses. CLAO J 1993;19:73.

Matthews TD, Frazer DG, Minassian DC, et al. Risk of keratitis and patterns of use with disposable contact lenses. Arch Ophthalmol 1992;110:1559.

Poggio EC, Abelson M. Complications and symptoms in disposable extended wear lenses compared with conventional soft daily wear and soft extended wear lenses. CLAO J 1993;19:31.

Poggio EC, Glynn RJ, Schein OD, et al. The incidence of ulcerative keratitis among users of daily-wear and extended-wear soft contact lenses. N Engl J Med 1989;321:779.

Sakamoto R, Miyanaga Y, Hamano H. Soft and RGP lens corneal swelling and deswelling with overnight wear. Int Contact Lens Clin 1991;18:214.

Schein OD, Glynn RJ, Poggio EC, et al. The relative risk of ulcerative keratitis among users of daily-wear and extended-wear soft contact lenses. A case control study. N Engl J Med 1989;321:773.

Solomon OD, Freeman MI, Boshnick EL, et al. A 3-year prospective study of the clinical performance of daily disposable contact lenses with frequent replacement and conventional daily wear contact lenses. CLAO J 1996;22:4.

Stapleton F, Dart J, Minassian D. Nonulcerative complications of contact lens wear. Relative risk for different lens types. Arch Ophthalmol 1992;110:1601.

Tsubota K, Yamada M. Corneal epithelial alterations induced by disposable contact lens wear. Ophthalmology 1992;99:1193.

9

Ocular Surface Immune Reactions and Contact Lens Wear

Bryan M. Gebhardt and Hikaru Hamano

Immunopathologic consequences of contact lens wear include giant papillary conjunctivitis, allergic conjunctivitis, cell-mediated hypersensitivity, and others. For the most part, these reactions generally are thought to be the result of host responses to endogenously or exogenously acquired deposits on the surface of the lenses. Just as allergists counsel their patients to avoid coming into contact with the allergen to which they are sensitive, eye care professionals must advise their contact lens patients that it is essential to keep their lenses clean to avoid these immune reactions. With the variability in allergic sensitivities and tendencies to deposit formation, however, even the most rigorous cleaning regimens can fail to prevent unwanted immune reactions that make contact lens wear difficult or impossible for some patients.

In this chapter, we present information regarding possible sources of antigenic substances on contact lenses, consider the potential for the development of immunity to such substances, and summarize possible therapeutic approaches to preventing such immunologic reactions.

TYPES OF IMMUNE REACTIONS

In the early 1960s, Gell and Coombs (1963) proposed a classification system for immunologic reactions. In this system, type 1 (allergic) hypersensitivity is synonymous with immediate hypersensitivity reactions (*antibody-mediated reactions*) mediated by antibodies of the immunoglobulin E (IgE) class and various low–molecular-weight mediators, such as histamines, platelet-activating factor, and serotonin. The conjunctival allergic reactions that occur in patients experiencing contact lens wear–related allergic hypersensitivity and patients with allergic conjunctivitis caused by such exogenous allergens as plant pollens are IgE-mediated hypersensitivity reactions.

Type 2 hypersensitivity, also referred to as *cytotoxic hypersensitivity* or *complement-dependent hypersensitivity*, is mediated by antibodies of the immunoglobulin classes other than IgE, including immunoglobulin M (IgM) and certain subclasses of immunoglobulin G (IgG). Type 3 hypersensitivity is synonymous with immune complex–mediated immunopathologic reactions. Antibodies combine with their antigens

175

to form large macromolecular complexes that activate the complement system, resulting in the release of vasoactive mediators, chemotactic substances, and cytotoxins that initiate inflammatory reactions and local cell death. There is no compelling evidence that either type 2 or type 3 hypersensitivity plays a role in any of the immune reactions seen in contact lens wearers.

Type 4 hypersensitivity, termed *delayed-type hypersensitivity* or *cell-mediated immunity*, is the function of thymus-derived lymphocytes (T lymphocytes or T cells). T cells recognize antigens, undergo blast transformation, divide, and secrete a variety of cytokines that result in the activation of immune effector cells, including macrophages, B lymphocytes (B cells), Langerhans' cells, and others. For example, T cells mediate the classic delayed-type hypersensitivity reaction seen in the skin of patients given intradermal injections of tuberculin, and this reaction is considered the prototypical type 4 hypersensitivity reaction.

Type 4 or cell-mediated hypersensitivity reactions may occur in contact lens wearers when self-proteins undergo denaturation as they are adsorbed onto the surface of the contact lens and then are recognized by T cells as nonself. This type of reaction may occur also in response to exogenous antigenic molecules that sensitize T cells. Environmental antigens in the form of foreign protein molecules and even very small organic molecules, such as substituted benzene ring compounds and other low–molecular-weight compounds, may link up with larger endogenous or self-protein molecules on corneal and conjunctival epithelial cell membranes. This linkage forms a relationship referred to as a *hapten-carrier* relationship. The hapten is the foreign molecule and the carrier is the self molecule; the carrier facilitates the presentation of the nonself hapten to the T cells, resulting in the production of antibody to the hapten and T cells that are sensitized specifically to that hapten. In contact lens wearers, the offending antigenic substances activate T cells that, in turn, secrete mediators that attract and stimulate a full range of effector cells, including macrophages, Langerhans' cells, histiocytes, basophils, and mast cells. The result of this type of reaction may be the progressive development of such immunologically mediated complications as giant papillary conjunctivitis or allergic conjunctivitis.

Thus, of the four types of hypersensitivity reactions, types 1 and 4 are those that may occur in contact lens wearers in response to exogenous stimuli, including environmental pollutants, medications, and additives to contact lens storage and cleaning solutions, and to endogenous stimuli (e.g., protein molecules adsorbed to contact lenses during wear).

CAUSES OF OCULAR SURFACE IMMUNE REACTIONS

Tear Protein Deposits

The tears provide the primary source of in vivo self-protein that can adsorb to contact lenses. The tear protein content at the ocular surface in the normal human eye ranges from 6 to 20 g/liter (Van Haeringen 1981). The predominant normal tear proteins are albumin and lysozyme. Also present are low concentrations of lactoferrin, immunoglobulin, and various complement components, as well as very low concentrations of other serum proteins, including transferrin, ceruloplasmin, and some enzymes (e.g., lactic dehydrogenase, glycolytic enzymes, amylase, peroxidase, and collagenase). The natural proteins themselves present no significant immunologic threat; in the process of adsorption to the surface of the contact lens,

Table 9.1 Properties of Hydrogel Lenses

Water Content (%)	Composition	Ionic or Nonionic
72	Dimethyl acrylamide (DMAA)	Nonionic
58	2-Hydroxyethyl methacrylate–methacrylic acid (HEMA-MA)	Ionic
38	2-Hydroxyethyl methacrylate (HEMA)	Nonionic

Source: Adapted from H Hamano, S Mitsunaga, M Moriyama, et al. Protein adsorption to hydrogel lenses. J Jpn Contact Lens Soc 1993;35:213.

however, they may be altered and denatured sufficiently so as to become recognizable by the immune system as nonself.

The immune response to these antigenic proteins could take the form of an antibody-mediated response (type 1), a cell-mediated response (type 4), or both. An antibody-mediated response could produce the signs and symptoms of allergic conjunctivitis, followed by a cellular conjunctivitis in the form of giant papillary conjunctivitis-like reactions. A cell-mediated response could cause a local chronic inflammatory reaction characterized by the infiltration of neutrophils; mast cells; Langerhans' cells; and other mononuclear cell types, including lymphocytes and macrophages. The ensuing tissue alteration and inflammation could result in tissue edema, abnormal tear production, and contact lens intolerance. Such immunopathologic reactions may be either acute or chronic and can be sufficiently uncomfortable to cause a patient to discontinue contact lens wear.

To examine the potential for variability in the formation of tear protein deposits on contact lenses made from different materials, Hamano et al. (1993) performed in vitro and in vivo studies of protein adsorption to three types of hydrogel lenses having different ionicities, water contents, and chemical compositions (Table 9.1).

In Vitro Studies of Tear Protein Deposits on Three Types of Contact Lenses

For the in vitro studies, a solution simulating tears (containing lysozyme, albumin, and immunoglobulin at a total final concentration of 7 g/liter) was prepared in physiologic saline. Each lens was immersed in an aliquot of the tear solution for a specified period of time, after which the lens was removed and placed in a sterile physiologic saline without tear proteins for the same period of time to permit elution of the proteins from the lenses. In all, each lens was eluted in two 1-ml portions of physiologic saline and then in two 1-ml portions of physiologic saline containing 1% sodium dodecylsulfate (SDS), a nonionic detergent. At the end of the elution period, the amount of protein in the solutions was determined by protein assay according to the method described by Bradford (1976).

The results indicate that the ionic, 58%-water-content hydroxyethyl methacrylate/methacrylic acid (HEMA-MA) lenses adsorbed the largest amount of protein, compared with the nonionic 72%-water-content dimethyl acrylamide (DMAA) lenses and the nonionic 38%-water-content hydroxyethyl methacrylate (HEMA) lenses, regardless of the length of the immersion in the tear solution (Table 9.2). Furthermore, although considerable protein was eluted from the HEMA-MA lenses in the saline solution alone, even larger amounts were eluted in the saline-detergent solution. In contrast, only small amounts of protein were eluted from the DMAA and

Table 9.2 Protein Adsorption to Hydrogel Lenses In Vitro

| Type of Lens | Incubation Time (min) | Protein (µg) Eluted | | |
		Saline	SDS-Saline	Total
72% DMAA	10	10	1	11
	30	19	0	19
	60	26	5	31
	120	7	4	11
	240	13	2	15
58% HEMA-MA	10	69	102	171
	30	103	149	252
	60	121	168	289
	120	167	232	399
	240	212	303	515
38% HEMA	10	11	1	12
	30	14	0	14
	60	18	1	19
	120	19	1	20
	240	20	0	20

SDS = sodium dodecylsulfate; DMAA = dimethyl acrylamide; HEMA-MA = 2-hydroxyethyl methacrylate methacrylic acid; HEMA = 2-hydroxyethyl methacrylate.
Note: Percentages refer to water content of lens material.
Source: Adapted from H Hamano, S Mitsunaga, M Moriyama, et al. Protein adsorption to hydrogel lenses. J Jpn Contact Lens Soc 1993;35:213.

HEMA lenses, and virtually all of that was obtained in the initial saline extraction, with very little remaining to be eluted in the saline-detergent solution. These in vitro results suggest that the nonionic DMAA and HEMA lenses may be less likely than the ionic HEMA-MA lenses to adsorb tear proteins in vivo and that adsorbed protein is removed much more readily from the nonionic lenses with standard cleaning solutions such as water or balanced salt solution.

In Figure 9.1, these data are plotted to show the kinetics of the adsorption of tear proteins in vitro. The ionic HEMA-MA lenses rapidly adsorbed protein, with significant quantities bound to the lenses within 10 minutes of immersion in the tear solution and adsorption continuing throughout the 4-hour incubation period. In contrast, the nonionic HEMA and DMAA lenses adsorbed very little protein from the tear solution over the total incubation time; the small amount of adsorption that did take place occurred within the first 10 minutes of immersion, with a steady-state level being maintained thereafter.

In Vivo Studies of Tear Protein Deposits on Three Types of Contact Lenses

In the in vivo studies, the DMAA and HEMA lenses were compared for their capacity to adsorb protein when worn on normal human eyes for periods of 6 and 24 hours (Table 9.3). As in the in vitro studies, the ionic contact lenses adsorbed the largest amount of tear proteins, and the nonionic lenses adsorbed much smaller amounts.

In the second part of the in vivo studies, the relationship between protein content in human tears and protein adsorption to the contact lens in the eye was examined. Tear samples were collected from patients before contact lens wear, and the protein con-

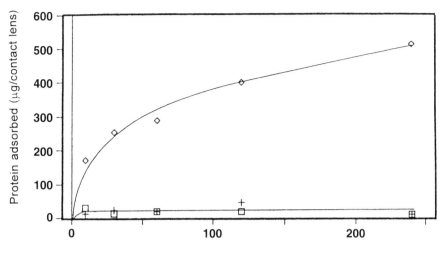

Duration of immersion in simulated tear solution (minutes)

Figure 9.1 The relationship between the amount of protein adsorbed and the duration of immersion in a solution containing tear proteins. ($\Diamond$ = ionic lenses with 58% water content; + = nonionic lenses with 72% water content; $\square$ = nonionic lenses with 38% water content. (Reprinted from H Hamano, S Mitsunaga, M Moriyama, et al. Protein adsorption to hydrogel lenses. J Jpn Contact Lens Soc 1993;35:213.)

Table 9.3 Protein Adsorption to Hydrogel Lenses In Vivo

Type of Lens	Duration of Lens Wear (hrs)	Protein (µg) Eluted		
		Saline	SDS-Saline	Total
72% DMAA	6	7	0	7
	24	12	9	21
58% HEMA-MA	6	115	190	305
	24	228	409	637

SDS = sodium dodecyl sulfate; DMAA = dimethyl acrylamide; HEMA-MA = 2-hydroxyethyl methacrylate methacrylic acid.
Note: The lenses were worn for the lengths of time indicated and eluted in two 1-ml volumes of saline and SDS-saline. Percentages refer to water content of lens material.
Source: Adapted from H Hamano, S Mitsunaga, M Moriyama, et al. Protein adsorption to hydrogel lenses. J Jpn Contact Lens Soc 1993;35:213.

centrations in the samples were compared with the amount of protein adsorbed by individual ionic and nonionic contact lenses after 6 and 24 hours of lens wear. As was the case in the in vitro studies, the ionic lenses adsorbed markedly more protein (Figure 9.2) than did the nonionic lenses (Figure 9.3). In general, more protein was adsorbed over the longer (24-hour) wearing period, compared with the shorter (6-hour) wearing period for both types of lenses. There appears to be no direct relationship, however, between the amount of protein in the tear sample from a given eye and the amount of protein adsorption (deposit formation) on the lenses worn by that eye.

On the basis of these studies, it appears that the ionic HEMA-MA contact lens has a much higher adsorptive affinity for tear proteins compared with the nonionic

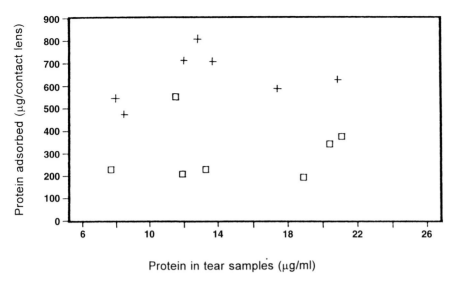

Figure 9.2 Ionic lenses (58%-water-content hydroxyethyl methacrylate-methacrylic acid). The amount of protein eluted from lenses worn for 6 or 24 hours was determined and plotted against the amount of protein in tear samples taken from the same eyes before contact lens wear.(□ = 6 hours; + = 24 hours.) (Reprinted from H Hamano, S Mitsunaga, M Moriyama, et al. Protein adsorption to hydrogel lenses. J Jpn Contact Lens Soc 1993;35:213.)

DMAA and HEMA lenses. Even the nonionic lenses were subject to protein adsorption to some degree, however, and the amount of protein adsorption on both types of lenses was quite variable from individual to individual. As discussed earlier in the section on tear protein deposits, if tear proteins become denatured in the course of adsorption to *any* lens, they could provide sufficient antigenic stimulation to lead to immunologic sensitization and the development of an immunopathologic disorder of the ocular surface that precludes contact lens wear.

Contact Lens Storage and Cleaning Solutions

The ingredients in lens storage solutions and lens cleaning solutions are a common source of potential allergens. As of this writing, these solutions are made up of sterile physiologic balanced salt solution, with such preservatives as polyaminopropyl biguanide or polyethylene glycol and occasionally including dilute solutions of detergents, such as Tween-20 or SDS. Compounds such as chlorhexidine and thimerosal have been found to cause adverse reactions in some patients. Although ocular sensitivity to chlorhexidine occurs in less than 1% of patients, this compound and others like it that can combine with self-carrier proteins on ocular surface cells and elicit immune reactions tend not to be used in cleaning and storage solutions for soft lenses.

Some contact lens cleaning solutions contain enzymes that function to remove or minimize protein deposits on the lens surfaces. One such enzyme, papain, was found to elicit allergic reactions in some lens wearers (Kaufman 1979). Again, there is a trend toward eliminating enzymes that cause allergic reactions and substituting newer molecules, such as subtilisin, that do not seem to be associated with adverse allergic phenomena in contact lens wearers.

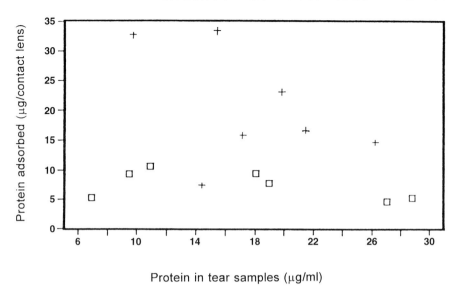

Figure 9.3 Nonionic lenses (72%-water-content dimethyl acrylamide). The amount of protein eluted from lenses worn for 6 or 24 hours was determined and plotted against the amount of protein in tear samples taken from the same eyes before contact lens wear. (□ = 6 hours; + = 24 hours.) (Reprinted from H Hamano, S Mitsunaga, M Moriyama, et al. Protein adsorption to hydrogel lenses. J Jpn Contact Lens Soc 1993;35:213.)

In principle, the mechanisms involved in the initiation of an allergic reaction at the ocular surface by the binding of reactive organic constituents of preservatives and contact lens cleansing solutions to cell surface protein molecules would be similar to those of the general immune response. For example, chlorhexidine or a constituent of thimerosal preservative solutions could bind to the cell surface proteins of conjunctival cells, corneal epithelial cells, or both. These complexes then could be presented to and recognized by cells of the immune system. Activation and sensitization of immunologically competent lymphocytes in the conjunctival-associated lymphoid tissue could result in the proliferation of these immune cells, stimulation of the production of antibodies specific for the eliciting antigen, and the production of cytokines by T cells. Antibodies directed against the nonself foreign preservative substances could bind to these substances, initiate inflammatory reactions mediated by the serum complement system, and precipitate classic inflammatory reactions in the conjunctiva and cornea. Mast cells and acute inflammatory cells would be attracted by chemotactic substances released as a consequence of the antigen-antibody-complement interactions, leading to tissue damage and conjunctivitis and ultimately to contact lens intolerance in the patient. This cycle of immunopathology usually is reversible and may be alleviated by changes in contact lens use, changes in contact lens cleaning solutions, and perhaps, for a time, abstinence from contact lens wear.

Contact Lens Materials and Additives

Contact lens manufacturers are well aware of the potential problems presented by additives used to stabilize and extend the shelf life of the contact lenses themselves and by additives incorporated into the lens matrix—additives that may leach out and be toxic or harmful to the lens wearer. The chemical formulations of all contact lenses are tested for toxicity before being used to prepare lenses for human use. Lenses prepared from DMAA, HEMA, and MA have been shown to be inert and nontoxic for human ocular surface cells. Lenses prepared from these polymers do not, over time, release breakdown products that are either antigenic or overtly toxic to the ocular surface.

The lens material appears to influence the formation of deposits of endogenous molecules, however. As seen in the studies by Hamano et al. (1993) described earlier, tear protein deposits appear to be a much more serious problem with lenses made from ionic polymers, and therefore the potential for denatured proteins eliciting an immune response may be a greater risk with these lenses.

PREVENTION OF IMMUNE RESPONSES RELATED TO CONTACT LENS WEAR

Probably the most severe immune reaction to contact lens wear is giant papillary conjunctivitis, characterized by the presence of giant papillae on the upper tarsal conjunctiva, mild itching, increased mucus secretion by the conjunctiva, and generalized ocular irritation. The genesis of this condition is not well understood. Hard lenses seem to be associated with a lower incidence of giant papillary conjunctivitis than are soft lenses, although any type of lens can cause this problem. The differential between the frequency of conjunctivitis in soft and hard contact lens wearers is not great, however, and the precise immunologic nature of the condition has not been established.

Generally, this disorder is classified as an immunologic reaction because of the histopathologic nature of the lesion and the symptomatology that is presented to the clinician (Allansmith et al. 1972). As previously suggested, either a cell-mediated hypersensitivity reaction (characterized by the infiltration of macrophages, histiocytes, and perhaps mast cells) or an antibody-mediated reaction (consisting of IgE-class antibodies directed against the offending antigens), or both, may play a role. A mixed reaction would help explain the histopathologic appearance of the giant papillae, including the presence of chronic inflammatory cells, mast cells, and other inflammatory components.

Recent reviews of this disorder include a comprehensive overview detailing a variety of clinical studies (Donshik 1994) and a succinct literature review and discussion of the association between giant papillary conjunctivitis and contact lens type, material, and deposits (Meisler and Keller 1995). Donshik (1994) hypothesizes that antigen deposits on contact lenses initiate a mixed cellular (type 4) and humoral (type 1) immune response resulting in the collection of inflammatory cells and mediators in the conjunctiva. Treatment of patients with ocular allergic symptoms, giant papillary conjunctivitis, or both would involve efforts to minimize antigen deposition and the use of mast cell stabilizers and nonsteroidal anti-inflammatory drugs to break the cycle of allergy and inflammation. Meisler and Keller (1995) raise the issue of a possible mechanical etiology and signal the importance of recognizing the possibility of a mixed origin involving local trauma and immune or inflammatory responses. Here again, the therapy would involve alleviation of the symptoms and drug treatment to interrupt the cycle of production of inflammatory mediators. Although it is clear that the exact cause is not yet known, it is generally concluded that treatment and prevention of recurrence must involve elimination of the stimulatory factors, which can be accomplished in a variety of ways, including careful attention to lens hygiene, topical drug therapy, and changing the type of lens worn or pattern of wear.

Lens Hygiene

Given that a major stimulatory factor is the presence of deposits on the lens surfaces, effective prevention requires regular and careful attention to lens cleaning. The eye care professional can make a major contribution to this effort with advice and support, but ultimately the burden of contact lens hygiene rests with the patient. Patients should be encouraged to report early symptoms of ocular surface abnormalities, such as allergic conjunctivitis or giant papillary conjunctivitis, at which time the ocular surface should be examined carefully, and the patient's habits regarding contact lens cleaning and wear should be reviewed.

Probably the best therapy for breaking a cycle of immunopathologic acute or chronic inflammatory ocular surface disease is to discontinue contact lens wear until the reaction subsides. Then, on resumption of contact lens wear, the patient should be followed carefully, and he or she should be provided with clear guidelines regarding maintenance and use of contact lenses. The eye care professional can recommend changes in contact lens use and wearing schedules; changes in contact lens storage, cleaning solutions, or both; and changes in patterns of behavior that may minimize or eliminate completely the conjunctivitis in most patients. Daily-disposable lenses should, at least theoretically, minimize the problem, although definitive data are not yet available.

Topical Drug Therapy

For patients who have chronic reactive problems due to contact lens wear, more drastic approaches may be necessary. It has been reported that topical corticosteroids, such as dexamethasone and prednisolone, cause the ocular inflammation to subside, but the chronic use of steroids has not been found to be uniformly beneficial in controlling giant papillary conjunctivitis (Allansmith et al. 1978; Kaufman 1979; Donshik et al. 1984).

Nonsteroidal anti-inflammatory agents have been tested as topical ocular preparations in a variety of conditions and may be of some value in treating or inhibiting the development of giant papillary conjunctivitis (Donshik et al. 1984; Wood et al. 1988). Nonsteroidal agents such as ketorolac and a variety of prostaglandin synthesis inhibitors (e.g., diclofenac and flurbiprofen) currently are being used for the treatment of giant papillary conjunctivitis secondary to extended contact lens wear.

Because a component of the ocular surface immune reactions generated during contact lens wear may be an allergic phenomenon, mast cell degranulation inhibitors, such as sodium cromolyn, have been used to treat affected patients (Meisler et al. 1982; Allansmith and Ross 1986; Kruger et al. 1992). These drugs inhibit the release of vasoactive, chemotactic, and inflammatory mediators by mast cells that have been triggered by IgE-class antibodies bound to the allergens. The ultimate value of these inhibitors in the treatment of contact lens–associated ocular inflammation and giant papillary conjunctivitis remains to be determined.

Changing the Type of Lens and the Pattern of Lens Wear

In general, if none of these approaches alleviate the patient's symptoms, it becomes necessary to suspend contact lens wear for a period of at least 2 weeks. Such patients then may be fitted with different soft contact lenses. Hard lenses also can be used if the patient can tolerate them and if they are cleaned scrupulously and carefully on a daily basis. Soft lenses made from different materials may be tried.

Disposable Lenses

A new approach to patients with intractable allergic reactions is the use of disposable lenses. In particular, daily-disposable lenses, worn for 1 day and discarded each night, may be an ideal solution because the short-term wear schedule eliminates the problems associated with removal of protein deposits on the lens surfaces. Because the patient puts a brand new lens on the eye each day, the potential for protein buildup is reduced, and the development of hypersensitivity reactions is unlikely. In such cases, however, the eye care professional must caution the patient strongly that attempting to economize by using the lenses for more than the prescribed 1-day wearing period will almost certainly result in a recurrence of the problem.

It is of some interest and curiosity that the papules that appear in giant papillary conjunctivitis can persist for months or longer, even after the patient becomes asymptomatic. Such patients may never be able to tolerate contact lenses. Thus, a very few patients may have to discontinue all lens use; for them, a return to spectacle correction or the possibility of refractive surgery may be the only alternatives.

REFERENCES

Allansmith MR, Ross RN. Ocular allergy and mast cell stabilizers. Surv Ophthalmol 1986;30:229.

Allansmith MR, Korb DR, Greiner JV. Giant papillary conjunctivitis induced by hard or soft contact lens wear: quantitative histology. Trans Am Acad Ophthalmol Otolaryngol 1978;85:766.

Allansmith MR, Korb DR, Greiner JV, et al. Giant papillary conjunctivitis in contact lens wearers. Am J Ophthalmol 1972;83:697.

Bradford MM. A rapid and sensitive method for the quantitation of microgram quantities of protein utilizing the principle of protein-dye binding. Anal Biochem 1976;72:248.

Donshik PC. Giant papillary conjunctivitis. Trans Am Ophthalmol Soc 1994;92:687.

Donshik PC, Ballow M, Luistro A, Samartine L. Treatment of contact lens-induced giant papillary conjunctivitis. CLAO J 1984;10:346.

Gell PGH, Coombs RRA. Clinical Aspects of Immunology. Oxford: Blackwell, 1963;317.

Hamano H, Mitsunaga S, Moriyama M, et al. Protein adsorption to hydrogel lenses. J Jpn Contact Lens Soc 1993;35:213.

Kaufman HE. Problems associated with prolonged wear of soft contact lenses. Ophthalmology 1979;86:411.

Kruger CJ, Ehlers WH, Luistro AE, Donshik PC. The treatment of giant papillary conjunctivitis with cromolyn sodium. CLAO J 1992;18:46.

Meisler DM, Keller WB. Contact lens type, material, and deposits and giant papillary conjunctivitis. CLAO J 1995;21:77.

Meisler DM, Berzins VJ, Krachmer JH. Cromolyn treatment of giant papillary conjunctivitis. Arch Ophthalmol 1982;100:1608.

Van Haeringen NJ. Clinical biochemistry of tears. Surv Ophthalmol 1981;26:84.

Wood TS, Stewart RH, Bowman RW, et al. Suprofen treatment of contact lens–associated giant papillary conjunctivitis. Ophthalmology 1988;95:822.

10

Keratitis and Contact Lenses

Herbert E. Kaufman

The list of complications occurring with the use of contact lenses is extensive (Smith and MacRae 1989; Stapleton et al. 1992). Corneal abrasions are nearly ubiquitous; it is a rare patient who has worn contact lenses over a period of years and has never had an abrasion. Some degree of corneal vascularization, especially encroaching on the limbus, is common in soft contact lens wearers, and recurring small areas of staining (epithelial ulcers) at 3 and 9 o'clock on the cornea are well-documented in hard contact lens wearers. Prolonged contact lens wear also can cause hypertrophic epithelium, with the production of abnormal basement membrane material, and can mimic carcinoma in situ. Giant papillary conjunctivitis can limit lens wear, and deposits of all sorts can be found on the lenses and are difficult to remove or prevent. The lenses themselves may be invaded by microorganisms. Of all of the complications of contact lens wear, however, the most devastating and most likely to cause visual loss is infectious keratitis (Smith and MacRae 1989).

Ulcerative keratitis, as defined by a loss of epithelium and an infiltrate in the stroma, is often difficult to diagnose and manage. Organisms can be cultured from a majority of these patients, but most studies indicate that between one-third and one-half of these specimens yield no organisms on culture. The small, round infiltrates are more common among contact lens wearers and must be treated as if they were infectious because true infection tends to spread so rapidly.

SYSTEMIC AND BEHAVIORAL FACTORS

A number of systemic and behavioral factors other than lens hygiene have been examined for their influence on the development of infectious keratitis (Schein et al. 1989). The only systemic condition found to be associated with increased risk was diabetes. Smoking also seemed to cause a moderate increase in the risk of ulcerative keratitis. Among the factors found to be unimportant were whether the lenses were the user's first pair, the age of the lenses, how often the lenses were worn while swimming or using a hot tub, and the length of time since the user had seen an eye care professional.

185

Table 10.1 Estimated Relative Risks of Ulcerative Keratitis with Daily-Wear and Extended-Wear Lenses Worn Overnight

Lens Type and Pattern of Use	Case Patients Versus Population-Based Controls	95% CI	*P* Value	Case Patients Versus Hospital-Based Controls	95% CI	*P* Value
Daily-wear						
No overnight use	1.00*	—	—	1.00*	—	—
Overnight use	8.96	4.09–19.63	.0001	9.55	2.87–31.80	.0002
Extended-wear						
No overnight use	2.76	1.06–7.20	.038	2.57	0.70–9.51	.156
Overnight use	10.17	5.29–19.55	.0001	15.04	5.21–43.43	.0001

CI = confidence interval.
*Standard against which other risks are defined.
Note: Case patients were 86 patients presenting with ulcerative keratitis associated with the use of soft contact lenses for cosmetic purposes. Two control groups were used: the population-based control group, consisting of 410 people who wore soft contact lenses for cosmetic purposes and who were identified by random telephone sampling, and the hospital-based control group, consisting of 61 people who wore soft contact lenses for cosmetic purposes and who presented to the participating eye clinics with acute ocular conditions unrelated to the use of contact lenses.
Source: Adapted from OD Schein, RJ Glynn, EC Poggio, et al. The relative risk of ulcerative keratitis among users of daily-wear and extended-wear soft contact lenses. A case-control study. N Engl J Med 1989;321:773.

OVERNIGHT WEAR AND CORNEAL ANOXIA

It is clear that the single most important factor in the development of infectious keratitis in contact lens wearers is overnight wear (Poggio et al. 1989; Schein et al. 1989, 1994; Smith and MacRae 1989). Wearing contact lenses overnight markedly increases the risk of infectious keratitis, and if the lenses are worn overnight for several consecutive nights, the risk is greater. For example, in a case-control study by Schein et al. (1989), users of extended-wear lenses who wore them overnight had a risk 10–15 times the risk of users of daily-wear lenses who did not wear them overnight (Table 10.1). Furthermore, daily-wear lens users who "sometimes" wore their lenses overnight had nine times the risk of users of the same lenses who did not wear them overnight. In a related population-based study by the same group (Poggio et al. 1989), the overall annualized incidence of ulcerative keratitis was estimated to be 4.1 per 10,000 persons per year using daily-wear soft contact lenses and more than five times as great (20.9 per 10,000 persons per year) for those using extended-wear soft contact lenses (Table 10.2).

The cause of increased risk of infectious keratitis may be multifactorial, but certainly there is evidence that oxygen deprivation is a major cause. It is clear that any lens now available worn on an extended-wear basis carries a significant additional risk of ulcerative keratitis, regardless of the type of lens (Poggio et al. 1989; Schein et al. 1989, 1994; Smith and MacRae 1989; MacRae et al. 1991). In rabbits, Solomon et al. (1994) showed that hypoxic corneal swelling is correlated with the risk of infection after contact lens wear if the eye is exposed to potentially pathogenic bacteria. In addition, however, they showed that any corneal epithelial damage, even without corneal

Table 10.2 Estimated Annualized Incidence of Ulcerative Keratitis per 10,000 Cosmetic Contact Lens Wearers and Estimated Relative Risk of Ulcerative Keratitis

Type of Lens	Incidence of Ulcerative Keratitis	95% CI	Relative Risk	95% CI
Daily-wear soft	4.1	2.9–5.2	1.00*	—
Extended-wear soft	20.9	15.1–26.7	5.15	3.47–7.65
Hard (PMMA)	2.0	0–4.4	0.50	0.15–1.65
Rigid gas-permeable	4.0	0–8.2	1.00	0.34–2.89

PMMA = polymethyl methacrylate; CI = confidence interval.
*Standard against which other risks are defined.
Source: Adapted from EC Poggio, RJ Glynn, OD Schein, et al. The incidence of ulcerative keratitis among users of daily-wear and extended-wear soft contact lenses. N Engl J Med 1989;321:779.

Table 10.3 Relative Rate of Formation of Corneal Ulcers in Patients for Daily and Extended Wear of Soft and Rigid Gas-Permeable Lenses

Comparison	Rate of Ulcer Formation
Type of wear	
Daily-wear	
Soft lenses vs. rigid gas-permeable lenses	1.00 : 1.29
Extended-wear	
Soft lenses vs. rigid gas-permeable lenses	1.00 : 1.31
Type of lens	
Soft	
Daily-wear vs. extended-wear	1.00 : 3.50
Rigid gas-permeable	
Daily-wear vs. extended-wear	1.00 : 3.50

Source: Adapted with permission from S MacRae, C Herman, RD Stulting, et al. Corneal ulcer and adverse reaction rates in premarket contact lens studies. Am J Ophthalmol 1991;111:457.

swelling, greatly increases the risk of infection. In a study from Cavanagh's laboratory, Imayasu et al. (1994) used confocal microscopy of rabbit eyes wearing rigid polymethyl methacrylate and gas-permeable lenses to demonstrate increasing areas of epithelial desquamation with decreasing oxygen permeability of the lens. They also showed that lactic dehydrogenase in the tears and bacterial adhesion seem to correlate with this phenomenon. The evidence was somewhat less convincing with soft contact lenses, however, in that there was no change in tear lactic dehydrogenase, less change in corneal swelling, and less epithelial desquamation, and no consideration was given to the biocompatibility of the various polymers.

As attractive as an anoxia hypothesis is, however, a number of findings seem not to support it. For instance, the risk of infectious keratitis is similar with daily wear of conventional polymethyl methacrylate hard lenses, rigid gas-permeable lenses, and soft lenses (see Table 10.2) (Poggio et al. 1989), and the risk of corneal ulcer is similar with extended wear of soft lenses and rigid gas-permeable lenses (Table 10.3) (MacRae et al. 1991). Even the rigid gas-permeable lenses with the highest oxygen permeability represent a significant risk of infection when worn overnight, and the risk is not much less than that of conventional soft contact lenses worn for a comparable period of time.

Other factors may also be involved. Changes in oxygen permeability are accompanied by changes in the lens polymers, and the interaction between the surface plastic of the contact lens and the surface of the eye may be critical. It also may be that at night, when tear flow is minimal and the eyes remain closed for long periods of time, what little tears are made run around the limbal gutter rather than over the corneal cap. Then the pressure of a contact lens on a relatively dry corneal apex, especially when accompanied by eye movement during REM (rapid eye movement) sleep, might induce microtrauma to the epithelium, leading to increased susceptibility to infection and ulcerative keratitis. (This would not play such a prominent role in rabbit studies because the rabbit blinks infrequently and its nictitating membrane usually is excised for the purposes of contact lens studies.) Further, Yamaguchi et al. (1984) suggested that the trapping of glucose and other metabolites within a soft contact lens might predispose to an invasion of the lens and that the higher the water content, the greater the possible risk. Biocompatibility factors also may play a role.

Whatever the factors involved in the increase in ulcerative keratitis with overnight wear, it is clear that any lens worn on an extended-wear basis carries a significant additional risk for ulcerative keratitis (Poggio et al. 1989; Schein et al. 1989, 1994; Smith and MacRae 1989; MacRae et al. 1991). It is important to recognize that no contact lens available today has been shown to be without risk when worn overnight. At the time of this writing, in the United States, the risk seems to be that 1 in every 300–450 extended-wear patients may develop ulcerative keratitis each year, and if the rate of infection remains constant over time, the risk will increase 10-fold for each decade of lens use (Poggio et al. 1989; Smith and MacRae 1989), so that over 10 years, it might be as high as 1 in 30.

It is also clear that removing the lens at night drastically reduces the risk of infectious keratitis, whatever type of lens is involved. Schein et al. (1994) estimated that 49–74% of contact lens–associated cases of ulcerative keratitis could be prevented by eliminating overnight wear. The convenience of extended-wear lens use is exquisite, but the risks, although modest, are real. At the time of this writing, these risks cannot be avoided by selecting any of the currently available lenses, even the very highly permeable rigid gas-permeable lenses.

CONTACT LENS CARE

Often, routine contact lens care is unsatisfactory, and this contributes to increased risk of infection with a variety of organisms. One study found that at least 50% of patients do not care for their lenses in an acceptably hygienic way (Donzis et al. 1987). Even when patients cleaned their lenses, they often neglected to clean the case in which the lenses were stored. Because amebas, bacteria, and fungi can live on the contact lens case and in any debris trapped in the case, cleaning the case seems to be at least as important as cleaning and disinfecting the lens. There is conflicting evidence about how important the hygiene of contact lenses is to the development of ulcerative keratitis, but present studies suggest that overnight wear is a far more important variable.

Acanthamoeba

Contact lens care is vitally important to prevent infection with *Acanthamoeba*. A few years ago, a tragic epidemic of amebic keratitis was traced largely to the use of

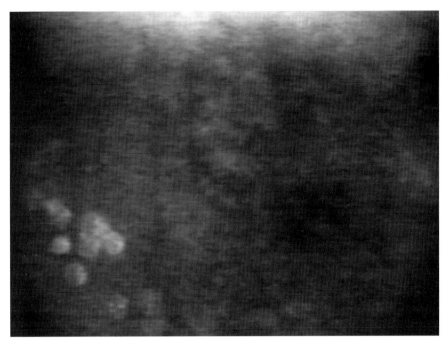

Figure 10.1 Confocal microscopy shows a cluster of *Acanthamoeba* cysts within the stroma of this patient. (Original magnification ×230.) (Courtesy of Stephen C. Kaufman, M.D., New Orleans, LA.)

unpreserved solutions for lens cleaning (Moore 1990). Even with the elimination of the use of salt tablets and tap water cleaning, however, amebic keratitis still occurs. Some cases can be traced to exposure to contaminated water (hot tubs, swimming pools, lakes, rivers, ponds, etc.), but for some, the source of the infection never is defined clearly. One case of amebic keratitis was reported in a patient who inserted a disposable soft contact lens directly from the manufacturer's package and neither removed nor manipulated the lens (Ficker et al. 1989), and we also have seen such a case. Disinfecting systems that can be used to kill *Acanthamoeba* include heat disinfection at 70–80°C for 10 minutes, 3% hydrogen peroxide for 2–3 hours, and 0.001% thimerosal with edetate for 4 hours. It should be noted, however, that except for heat disinfection, all the effective procedures require several hours, which tends to reduce compliance and increase the chance of infection.

Confocal Microscopy

Although it is not generally available clinically at the time of this writing, confocal microscopy seems to be by far the most sensitive and reliable approach to recognizing amebic keratitis (Kaufman et al. 1995). In vivo confocal microscopy of a cornea infected with *Acanthamoeba* can demonstrate either the trophozoite form or the cystic form of the organism. The trophozoite appears as an irregularly shaped, flattened, hyperreflective object that may resemble an elongated S. The cyst is recognized as a round or octagonal hyperreflective object within the cornea (Figure 10.1). Fungal keratitis also can be recognized reliably with this instrument. For instance, *Candida*, which is a yeast, appears primarily as fine, hyperreflective dots within the tissue,

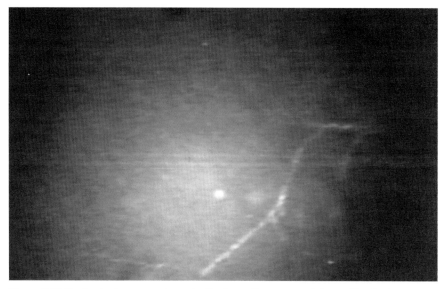

Figure 10.2 Confocal microscopy shows the fine branching pattern of *Aspergillus fumigatus* within the disrupted stroma of this patient. (Original magnification ×230.) (Courtesy of Stephen C. Kaufman, M.D., New Orleans, LA.)

whereas *Aspergillus* displays the fine branching pattern characteristic of this mold (Figure 10.2).

Dr. William Mathers, who has used confocal microscopy to examine ameba-infected corneas (Winchester et al. 1995), has suggested that, on the basis of his experience with clinical confocal microscopy, amebic keratitis may be far more common than was previously suspected and may be self-limiting in many cases. Where treatment is required, however, early recognition is important. In the early stages, amebic keratitis may resemble superficial epithelial ulceration, and if the ameba is recognized promptly, it is possible that epithelial debridement can prevent stromal invasion. Also, newer treatments, such as polyhexamethylene biguanide (Larkin et al. 1992; Mills et al. 1993; Varga et al. 1993), if used soon enough, seem to greatly improve the chance for success with medical therapy.

DISPOSABLE EXTENDED-WEAR LENSES

The hazards of overnight wear combined with the proven lack of compliance with lens hygiene recommendations create a real but potentially avoidable danger. As one approach to solving the problem of lens hygiene, disposable extended-wear contact lenses seemed attractive. However, although there are some conflicting data, most studies indicate that disposable lenses worn overnight for a period of 1–2 weeks do not decrease the risk of complications. The risks inherent in overnight wear far outweigh any possible gain from improved hygiene, and studies have shown that disposable soft contact lens wearers wearing their lenses overnight have a 14–16 times greater risk of developing ulcerative keratitis than daily-wear soft or rigid gas-permeable lens wearers (Table 10.4) (Buehler et al. 1992; Matthews et al. 1992).

Table 10.4 Relative Risk of Disposable Contact Lens Wear

Type of Lens	Relative Risk	95% CI	Adjusted Risk	95% CI
Daily-wear soft	1.00[a]	—	1.00	—
Daily-wear rigid gas-permeable	0.86	0.27–2.74	0.90	0.28–2.93
Disposable extended-wear soft[b]	13.47	5.50–32.97	14.34	5.47–37.63

CI = confidence interval.
[a]Standard against which other risks are defined.
[b]Disposable extended-wear lenses were worn for an average of 6 days (range of 1–8 days). Adjusted risk is adjusted for age and sex.
Source: Adapted with permission from PO Buehler, OD Schein, JF Sampler, et al. The increased risk of ulcerative keratitis among disposable soft contact lens users. Arch Ophthalmol 1992;110:1555–1558. ©1992, American Medical Association.

DAILY-DISPOSABLE LENSES

The risk of ulcerative keratitis, and in fact corneal complications in general, can be minimized by daily removal of the lens. In addition, the risks of ineffective hygiene and possible contamination of the lens case (often not as easily cleaned as the lens) are avoidable with daily-disposable contact lenses. Thus, sterile daily-disposable lenses may solve the problems of both lens hygiene and the risk of overnight wear. Such lenses are provided in the manufacturer's sterile pack, are worn for 1 day, and are discarded daily. There is some risk that patients still might use these lenses for extended wear, but proper education may prevent this.

No daily-disposable lenses with high oxygen permeability are available now, but none of the reported studies to date have shown an association between oxygen permeability and ulcerative keratitis with daily wear. Although the balance between safety, cost, and convenience still must be considered carefully, and the contact lens that is ideal for all patients has yet to be developed, there is no presently available lens that can be worn overnight as an extended-wear lens with the safety of a daily-wear lens. Based on studies available to date, daily-disposable lenses appear to provide the greatest safety of all.

REFERENCES

Buehler PO, Schein OD, Sampler JF, et al. The increased risk of ulcerative keratitis among disposable soft contact lens users. Arch Ophthalmol 1992;110:1555.

Donzis PB, Mondino BJ, Weissman BA, Bruckner DA. Microbial contamination of contact lens systems. Am J Ophthalmol 1987;104:325.

Ficker L, Hunter P, Seal D, Wright P. *Acanthamoeba* keratitis occurring with disposable contact lens wear. Am J Ophthalmol 1989;108:453.

Imayasu M, Petroll WM, Jester JV, et al. The relation between contact lens oxygen transmissibility and binding of *Pseudomonas aeruginosa* to the cornea after overnight wear. Ophthalmology 1994;101:371.

Kaufman SC, Laird J, Beuerman RW. In vivo, real-time confocal microscopy of fungal, bacterial, and *Acanthamoeba* keratitis [ARVO abstract]. Invest Ophthalmol Vis Sci 1995;36(suppl):S1022.

Larkin DFP, Kilvington S, Dart JKG. Treatment of *Acanthamoeba* keratitis with polyhexamethylene biguanide. Ophthalmology 1992;99:185.

MacRae S, Herman C, Stulting RD, et al. Corneal ulcer and adverse reaction rates in premarket contact lens studies. Am J Ophthalmol 1991;111:457.

Matthews TD, Frazer DG, Minassian DC, et al. Risks of keratitis and patterns of use with disposable contact lenses. Arch Ophthalmol 1992;110:1559.

Mills RA, Wilhelmus KR, Osato MS, Pyron M. Polyhexamethylene biguanide in the treatment of *Acanthamoeba* keratitis. Aust NZ J Ophthalmol 1993;21:277.

Moore MB. *Acanthamoeba* keratitis and contact lens wear. The patient is at fault. Cornea 1990;9(suppl):S33.

Poggio EC, Glynn RJ, Schein OD, et al. The incidence of ulcerative keratitis among users of daily-wear and extended-wear soft contact lenses. N Engl J Med 1989;321:779.

Schein OD, Buehler PO, Stamler JF, et al. The impact of overnight wear on the risk of contact lens–associated ulcerative keratitis. Arch Ophthalmol 1994;112:186.

Schein OD, Glynn RJ, Poggio EC, et al. The relative risk of ulcerative keratitis among users of daily-wear and extended-wear soft contact lenses. A case-control study. N Engl J Med 1989;321:773.

Smith RE, MacRae SM. Contact lenses—convenience and complications [editorial]. N Engl J Med 1989;321:824.

Solomon OD, Loff H, Perla B, et al. Testing hypotheses for risk factors for contact lens–associated infectious keratitis in an animal model. CLAO J 1994;20:109.

Stapleton F, Dart J, Minassian D. Nonulcerative complications of contact lens wear. Relative risks for different lens types. Arch Ophthalmol 1992;110:1601.

Varga JH, Wolf TC, Jensen HG, et al. Combined treatment of *Acanthamoeba* keratitis with propamidine, neomycin, and polyhexamethylene biguanide. Am J Ophthalmol 1993;115:466.

Winchester K, Mathers WD, Sutphin JE, Daley TE. Diagnosis of *Acanthamoeba* keratitis in vivo with confocal microscopy. Cornea 1995;14:10.

Yamaguchi T, Hubbard A, Fukushima A, et al. Fungus growth on soft contact lenses with different water contents. CLAO J 1984;10:166.

Index